Academic Ableism

Corporealities: Discourses of Disability

Series editors: David T. Mitchell and Sharon L. Snyder

A complete list of titles in the series can be found at www.press.umich.edu

Academic Ableism

Disability and Higher Education

JAY TIMOTHY DOLMAGE

University of Michigan Press
Ann Arbor

Published in the United States of America by the
University of Michigan Press
Manufactured in the United States of America
♾ Printed on acid-free paper

2020   2019   2018   2017   4   3   2   1

A CIP catalog record for this book is available from the British Library.

Library of Congress Cataloging-in-Publication data has been applied for.

ISBN 978–0-472–07371–9 (hardcover : alk. paper)
ISBN 978–0-472–05371–1 (paper : alk. paper)
ISBN 978–0-472–12341–4 (e-book)
http://dx.doi.org/10.3998/mpub.9708722

Cover description for accessibility: The cover features bold colors and bold,
oversize typography. Against a black background the word ACADEMIC is
written in white and the word ABLEISM in red. The cover is not wide enough
to accommodate the size of these words, so the words are intentionally
broken: ACA-, then below this DEMIC, then below this ABLE- and then ISM
(suggesting among other things that something in academia is broken). To the
left is a small photograph of the sculpture *Untitled* (Spiral Staircase) by Peter
Coffin. The sculpture consists of metal stairs that go nowhere, but instead
curve back into themselves in one continuous tangle. The author's name, Jay
Timothy Dolmage, appears in the top left corner; at the bottom of the page is
the subtitle of the book, DISABILITY AND HIGHER EDUCATION.

For Marilyn Dolmage, still building inclusive schools

Acknowledgments

———— ⚘ ————

Thanks to all of the folks who have shared their energy and dedication through the Committee on Disability Issues in College Composition over the years, from my mentor Cindy Lewiecki-Wilson to my first, finest, and continued coconspirators Stephanie Kerschbaum, Margaret Price, and Amy Vidali, through to all of those who will continue this work into the future.

Thanks to Brenda Brueggeman for tremendous, honest feedback. Thanks to the University of Michigan Press, the Editorial Board, and LeAnn Fields, for supporting not just the book but also its accessible delivery.

This book is intended to be useful to others, to make space for future advocacy and thinking, and to be built on, critiqued, and exceeded. Like most academic work, nothing here is truly mine, nothing truly new or original. This book is the product of learning with and from others. If I could, I'd list hundreds of coauthors, with my name last.

Contents

Introduction

The Approach

———— ❧ ————

John Dewey, the famous philosopher of education, in 1895:

"It is advisable that the teacher should understand, and even be able to criticize, the general principles upon which the whole educational system is formed and administered." (199)

As Ellen Cushman began writing about the "Rhetorician as Agent of Social Change," in her influential article about breaking down the barriers between universities and the communities around them, she first described the steep steps of "the Approach," a set of stairs, long in disrepair, between the city of Troy, New York, and Rensselaer Polytechnic Institute. The Approach, for her, symbolized that which "prohibit(s) scholars from Approaching people outside the University" (374). Every day, she writes, "we reproduce this distance so long as a select few gain entrance to universities, so long as we differentiate between experts and novices, and so long as we value certain types of knowledge we can capitalize on through specialization" (374). Here is a postcard picture of how the steps used to look (see page 2).

The steps are made of a light gray stone. They are about 20 meters wide on their bottom flight, which is at the forefront of the photo, so that we look up from the very bottom. The steps narrow further up, at the point where two large cylindrical marble columns stand. The steps con-

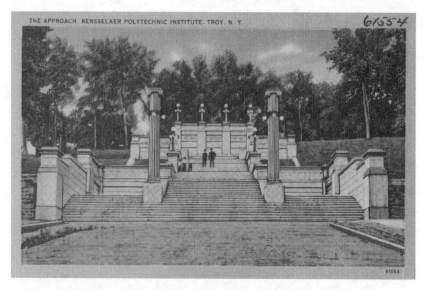

Fig. 1. "Postcard: Approach to Rensselaer." Rensselaer Polytechnic Institute
Library Archives, 1910.

tinue to climb up to an imposing set of gates. Behind these gates there
are green trees and foliage and, we assume, the university. Five people
stand up near the very top of the steps and they look very small, giving
perspective on just how steep and massive the approach is.

The very fact that these steps are featured in a postcard reveals the
ways that such structures are the stylistic and aesthetic center of many
campuses. If we were to object that such steps make the university inaccessible, many universities would make the argument that steep steps are
stylistically desirable, that they fit with the template, the architectural fingerprint of the school: all the buildings are the same color, with the same
size Ionic columns, maybe even the same number of stairs leading up to
buildings. These counterarguments show the ways that in the construction and maintenance of the steep steps there is also a latent argument
about aesthetics or appearances, one that trips over to the classroom,
into ideology and into pedagogy, where teachers are also sometimes concerned about pattern, clarity, propriety—and these things are believed
to be "beautiful" (access Hunter).[1] Today, the steps in this postcard are
in ruins, but the ideology of the steep steps persists, at Rensselaer and
elsewhere. Even as universities have become more accepting of diversity, academics tend to stay "inside," as Ellen Cushman suggests. And
the steps aren't the only way in which the university is inaccessible, even

if they might be the most physically arresting and apparent. As a select few stay in, disability is kept out, often quite literally. If it isn't the steep steps of this approach, it might be the ornate gates you encounter in the approach to Ivy League schools like Harvard and Princeton—gates that are reproduced in a movie like *Monsters University* as emblematic of college architecture and its ideology (more on this later).

Lower Education

Disability has always been constructed as the inverse or opposite of higher education. Or, let me put it differently: higher education has needed to create a series of versions of "lower education" to justify its work and to ground its exceptionalism, and the physical gates and steps trace a long history of exclusion.

For most of the 20th century, people with disabilities were institutionalized in asylums, "schools" for the "feeble-minded" and other exclusionary institutions, locations that became the dark shadows of the college or university, connected with residential schools, prisons, quarantines, and immigration stations in these shadows. These shadow locations also had steep steps and ornate gates, meant to hold the public out and to imprison people within, ensuring that the excluded couldn't mix with others within society; they were connected in a perverse way to the hope that the elite would mingle and mix with one another exclusively in colleges and universities. Further, the ethic of higher education still encourages students and teachers alike to accentuate ability, valorize perfection, and stigmatize anything that hints at intellectual (or physical) weakness.

In the early 1970s, David Rothman, a social historian of medicine, wrote a highly influential book called *The Discovery of the Asylum*. The book showed not just how asylums developed but how they allowed society to impose order through their connections with factories, hospitals, schools, and other institutions. When Rothman lists the similarities between the asylums, prisons, mental hospitals, reformatories, and almshouses developed in North America, he suggests that "there is a consensus among historians about their major characteristics":

> Confinement became the prime response to deviance;
> All of these places, regardless of their official function, adopted the same patterns and regimes of order and organization and they had a "unity of design and structure";

They were "in every sense apart from society";

"All of the institutional routines were segmented into carefully defined blocks of time, scrupulously maintained and punctuated by bells";

The routine was based on "work and solitude . . . steady labor and isolation" in which individuals are enveloped in the same work in a parallel way;

They began as orderly and eventually became overcrowded and corrupt;

They all housed the lowest orders of society. (xxv)

What is ironic about this list is that if you flip a few key points, you have a great description of the universities also being developed in the same period: fully removed, rigidly patterned, isolating, labor-intensive, increasingly corrupted and corruptible, but for only the highest orders of society. Perhaps the university should always have been thought of as similar to other "total institutions"—to borrow Erving Goffman's term. Perhaps the college or university is in fact exactly the same as the alms-house or asylum, organizationally and even architecturally. And yet it is viewed as the opposite. Thus the subjects in one total institution, the college, are elevated. The inmates in the other spaces are confined. Importantly: one studies; the other is studied.

As Sharon Snyder and David Mitchell have shown, "historically, disabled people have been the objects of study but not the purveyors of the knowledge base of disability" (Cultural, 198). As Tanya Titchkosky writes, "disabled people are socially organized under the rubric of knowledge bases . . . within the everyday practices and procedures of university environments, for example, [we think of] disability as a problem in need of a solution" and not as an "important form of critical knowledge production within the university" (Question, 70). Disability is studied; people with disabilities have been research resources. More than this, higher education has been built upon such research.

It is important to map the history of this research, but also to intervene in showing some of the ways that we might hope higher education can be redesigned. We need to understand how universities work to fully understand disability. Inversely, we really need to understand disability to understand the history and the future of higher education. To develop this understanding, I will build upon the crucial historical work of scholars such as Craig Steven Wilder, Heather Munro Prescott, and Christina Cogdell, who have revealed the racist, ableist, eugenicist roots of higher education. I will also build upon the crucial theoretical work of scholars such as Stephanie Kerschbaum, Tanya Titchkosky, Margaret Price, and Sara Ahmed who have revealed the racist, ableist, eugenic character of current academic culture. This research has allowed for an ongoing critique of the exclusive machinery of higher education and its physical, economic, affective (or emotional) costs. I will engage with all of this work carefully and extensively in this book. More broadly, this book will also bring together two specific academic fields or approaches: rhetoric and disability studies.

Disability Studies and Rhetoric

Disability studies is a field that has "emerged"—to borrow the words of one of its leading scholars, Rosemarie Garland-Thomson ("Disability Studies"). There are majors, minors, graduate programs, faculty positions, and departments of disability studies at colleges and universities. These departments almost always differentiate themselves from approaches to studying disability medically, or as subject to rehabilitation and therapy. This field of disability studies takes a critical approach to disability, grounded in disability rights and foregrounding the experiences and perspectives of people with disabilities, maintaining that disability is a political and cultural identity, not simply a medical condition.

Disability studies is an interdisciplinary, multidisciplinary field of study. Disability studies disrupts the idea that disabled people should be defined primarily through their disabilities by others, retaining instead the right for disabled people to define their own relationships with disability. As I have shown in other work, but also (more importantly) as has been shown within the field over decades of work, disability studies critiques representations of disability as pathology, as needing to be cured or killed or eradicated, as needing to be overcome or compensated for, as an object of pity or charity, as a sign of an internal flaw or a social ill or signal from above, as isolating, as a symptom of the abuse of nature, as existing on a continuum in which one disability is always accompanied by other disabilities or, conversely, in which some disabilities are clearly better than others. In the words of Danielle Peers and Joshua St. Pierre:

> Stories about us [disabled people] are boring. As predictable and ubiquitous as they are dangerous, normate narrations of our lives are as straight as they come: one-dimensional narratives of tragic loss

and/or progressive normativity. We are dying or overcoming. We become a burden or an inspiration. We desire vindication or marriage. Our entire narrative worlds are defined by our Otherness, yet revolve around the normates and the normative. These stories cut straight to the point, using—and used as—well-steeped, easily readable metaphors bolstered by the requisite piano-based musical cues. If we didn't know us better, we would bore us. (1)

As Lennard Davis and other disability studies scholars have pointed out, the categories of normal and abnormal, able and disabled are invented and enforced in service of "a certain kind of society," in service of particular ideologies (Enforcing, 9–11). This "certain type of society" or ableist "reality" that Davis alludes to has been created, and is maintained, through higher education. Further, as Douglas Baynton has written, "disability has functioned historically to justify inequality for disabled people themselves, but it has also done so for women and minority groups. . . . the concept of disability has been used to justify discrimination against other groups by attributing disability to them" (33). Again, higher education has been the place where the dividing lines of this discrimination have been decided. Thus, when Garland-Thomson suggests that disability studies has "emerged" as an academic discipline, this is a notable spatial metaphor. What disability studies has emerged out of are institutions in which disability as a negative concept, as a form of disqualification, was invented and applied and cemented. Even if disability studies has emerged, it has emerged only partially from within an architecture in which ableism has an incredibly powerful hold. In discussing this emergence, it is essential to understand that disability studies has emerged into higher education, the location so powerfully responsible for the suppression of disabled people. And if disability studies has emerged in academia, this emergence cannot overwrite the activist, community-based roots of the disability rights movement, even when these connections and roots are often ignored.

But let me pause here to define some terms. Because higher education employs logics of both *ableism* as well as *disablism*. "Disablism" can be defined as "a set of assumptions (conscious or unconscious) and practices that promote the differential or unequal treatment of people because of actual or presumed disabilities" (Kumari Campbell, 4). Disablism, in short, negatively constructs disability. Disablism negatively constructs both the values and the material circumstances around people with disabilities. Disablism says that there could be nothing worse than being disabled, and treats disabled people unfairly as a result of these values. Ableism, on the other hand, instead of situating disability as bad and focusing on that stigma, positively values able-bodiedness. In fact, ableism makes able-bodiedness and able-mindedness compulsory. Disablism constructs disability as negative quite directly and literally. Ableism renders disability as abject, invisible, disposable, less than human, while able-bodiedness is represented as at once ideal, normal, and the mean or default. The title of this book focuses on the term ableism not because disablism isn't present in higher education and academia—it absolutely is—and disablism can never be fully disconnected from ableism. But academia powerfully mandates able-bodiedness and able-mindedness, as well as other forms of social and communicative hyperability, and this demand can best be defined as ableism. In fact, few cultural institutions do a better or more comprehensive job of promoting ableism. What we also learn from higher education is that disablism is almost always wrapped into, and sometimes hidden within, ableism. That is, to value ability through something like the demand to overcome disability, or a research study to cure disability, there is also an implicit belief that being disabled is negative and to be avoided at all costs. This belief then leads to structures in which disabled people live in poverty, are underemployed, and so on. As activist and scholar Lydia Brown writes, "ableism is not some arbitrary list of 'bad words,' as much as language is a tool of oppression. Ableism is violence, and it kills" (n.p.).

The book then moves back and forth between a perspective from this "emergence" of disability studies, a perspective in which we can use disability studies to effectively critique education, and a perspective in which disability is still actively submerged or controlled within academia, in which there is no more ableist location than the university.

To facilitate this movement between spheres, it helps to bring disability studies together with rhetoric. Rhetoricians focus on the uses of language to persuade or to change people's actions and opinions. Most people think of rhetoric only in a negative sense—as the intentional misuse of language to mislead and misdirect. Yet rhetoricians recognize the ways that words and languages and meaning-making systems shape beliefs, values, institutions, and even bodies—sometimes negatively, sometimes positively, often powerfully. One simple way to define rhetoric is to say that it is the study of all of communication. But more specifically, rhetoricians foreground the persuasive potential of all texts, linking language to power. As Melanie Yergeau and John Duffy write in an article defining autism and rhetoric, "rhetoric functions as a powerfully shaping instrument for creating conceptions of identity and positioning individuals relative to established social and economic hierarchies. A function of the rhetorical scholar is to identify such powerfully shaping instruments and their effects upon individuals, including disabled individuals" (n.p.). As they argue, rhetoric is not only useful for studying disability, it is necessary, indispensable.

In previous work I have defined rhetoric as the strategic study of the circulation of power through communication (access Disability Rhetoric). Further, I believe that we should recognize rhetoric as the circulation of discourse through the body. This circulation takes on added meaning when we combine rhetorical study with what we might call "institutional critique" and with "rhetorical space." Institutions (and their geographies) are powerfully rhetorical, and this rhetorical power shapes the bodies within these spaces. Finally, then: colleges and universities are rhetorically constructed. It isn't necessary to be a rhetorician to understand this shaping. But all stakeholders in higher education can utilize rhetorical tools both to better understand academia and to change it.

James Porter, Patricia Sullivan, Stuart Blythe, Jeff Grabill, and Libby Meyers wrote about the rhetorical methodology they call institutional critique, a means of carefully interrogating how organizations are put together. They noted that "the materiality of institutions is constructed with the participation of rhetoric" (625, italics mine). One builds academia as one imagines its spaces. It follows that stakeholders can also "change disciplinary practices through the reform of institutional structures" (619). As Amy Wan shows (channeling philosopher John Dewey), the classroom is a "protopublic" space (31). This term means that the classroom shapes larger communities. There is tremendous potential, and tremendous responsibility, then, to examine these buildings we work in, and how they are involved in building a larger social and public space outside of these walls (and gates and stairs).

These institutional structures can then be understood through the lens of what feminist rhetorician Roxanne Mountford calls "rhetorical space." Mountford urges us to consider "the effect of physical spaces on communicative event[s]"; the ways that "rhetorical spaces carry the residue of history upon them, but also, perhaps, something else: a physical representation of relationships and ideas" (42). She argues that space "carries with it the sediment of cultural tradition, of the social imaginary" (63). Richard Marback builds on this argument, claiming that a location can be seen as a "nexus of cultural, historical, and material conditions" of oppression, and can become a "physical representation of . . . injustice" (1). Simply: one can read inequity and inequality in the buildings, patterns, and positions of the university. *Academic Ableism* will both study the university as a rhetorical space that holds a history of injustice in its architecture, but will also seek to reshape these spaces through critique, persuasion, and pedagogy. If rhetoric is the circulation of discourse through the body, then spaces and institutions cannot be disconnected from the bodies within them, the bodies they selectively exclude, and the bodies that actively intervene to reshape them.

Such an approach flips back and forth between physical space and rhetorical space. That is, while rhetorical space may take as its inspiration or focus actual physical structures, it extends these structures to better understand how they also discipline or influence ideas. Something like the steep stairs outside of a university lecture hall can be critiqued as a spatial and architectural feature that excludes; the stairs can also be understood as making a rhetorical argument or sending a message at the same time; and also at the very same time the stairs should push us to understand that other features of the institution that may not be as immediately recognizable to us, also set up steep steps—and these can range from the subject matter being spoken about in that lecture hall, to the rote, stand-and-deliver model of pedagogy and its toll on many students and many teachers, to the actual cost of being in that lecture hall in the first place. When we bring together a study of rhetorical space, institutional critique, and disability studies, we have to understand that all of these things as connected.

This connected reading shows that while the stairs may keep out certain bodies and exclude certain disabilities, institutions don't just make it hard to get around in wheelchairs or on crutches—though this is absolutely part of how academia excludes. Instead, physical inaccessibility is always linked—not just metaphorically—to mental, intellectual, social, and other forms of inaccessibility.

Disability studies scholars often show how disability is represented as a catch-all. People with physical disabilities are assumed to be cognitively disabled, representations of physical disability often rely on reinforcement from suggestions of mental or physical deficit, something we might call "disability drift" (access Dolmage, Disability Rhetoric). Drift is linked to the idea that some disabilities (i.e., physical disabilities) are better than others (i.e., mental or cognitive). On campus, this hierarchy is very real. To a certain degree, all disabilities on college campuses are invisible—until an accommodation is granted, they have no legal reality.

But so-called invisible disabilities are particularly fraught in an educational setting in which students with disabilities are already routinely and systematically constructed as faking it, jumping a queue, or asking for an advantage. The stigma of disability is something that drifts all over—it can be used to insinuate inferiority, revoke privilege, and step society very freely. But the legal rights that come with disability do not drift very easily at all.

Ableism drifts. Therefore, so must accommodations and access. When educators recognize physical inaccessibility, they can and should read intellectual and social inaccessibility into this space. We currently live in a society in which one single disability can be linked to any other disability in a negative way. But could we live in a society in which the accessibility we create for one person can also lead us to broaden and expand accessibility for all? On the way to this world, educators at least have to recognize that physical access is not "enough"—it is not where accessibility should stop.

Disability is also used to shore up other stigmatization—very importantly, the categories of gender, race, and sexuality have relied upon the attribution of biological inferiority, for instance. This is another way disability drifts. So I will be trying—very carefully—to show how academia has used ableism (and continues to use ableism) to marginalize specific groups of students.

It may seem problematic to group different disabilities and different communities of people with disabilities, including those who may be labeled or stigmatized, but don't claim disability identity (and may even disavow it). Certainly, perspectives on disability vary and are constantly contested. There are many different disabilities represented within disability studies—visible and invisible, physical and mental, et cetera and so on. There are tensions created by this grouping; and on the other hand the grouping constantly grows as new alliances and commonalities are found. Disability studies creates common ground in the experience of stigma and oppression, in the fight for more positive representations, and in the ongoing struggle for physical and intellectual access. In the end, what counts as a disability (and especially what does not) is of much greater interest to those who seek to criticize disability studies from outside of the field. Unfortunately, I will need to dig much more deeply into these accusations of "faking" disability throughout this book.

The goal here is not to deconstruct the concept of disability as it attaches to certain bodies by saying that this person or that group is not disabled. Instead, the goal is to affirm disability as a shared and positive identity, while challenging the use of disability as something that can be used to disqualify or stigmatize. We cannot recognize the foundations and futures of academia if we are constantly dodging the idea of disability. Instead, educators have to recognize these very foundations and futures as being built upon ableism, and as—literally—being built upon the bodies of disabled people.

Eugenics and Colonial Science

Another key term within the history of higher education is eugenics.

I define eugenics as the "science" of controlling who lives, who procreates, who thrives, and who dies, based on flawed ideas about our genetic makeup. For instance, as I have shown in other work, beginning at the turn of the twentieth century, eugenics characterized and drove North American national health and immigration policy. In addition to the "negative" eugenic programs of sterilization, lynching, and so on, carried out over decades across the country, immigration was ideal for "positive" eugenics, literally offering opportunities to control and edit the gene pool, using immigration stations as an elaborate sieve (access Dolmage, Disabled Upon Arrival). Eugenics led to practices and processes that selected and sorted bodies into geographical areas, classes, and regimes of discipline. Eugenics also inspired genocide. Eugenics was a philosophy, a dogma, a rhetoric, a religion.

Beginning at the turn of the twentieth century, eugenics was "anointed guardian of [American] health and character," as Nancy Ordover has shown (xiv). Historians have come to understand that eugenics was a powerful rhetoric as well as a series of practices. As L. Glenna Leland, Margaret A. Gollnick, and Stephen S. Jones show in their research on course offerings, the teaching of actual classes on eugenics, especially at larger land grant institutions, was widespread at North American schools, providing an "opportunity structure" for eugenics to become a widespread and transnational social movement. Simply, the teaching of eugenics at North American schools markedly sped the growth and popularity of the ideas. The authors go on to say that these "opportunity structures persisted even after eugenics faded as an international movement" following the Holocaust (67). In sociology, an "opportunity structure" names the conditions or factors that might empower people to create social movements. A university class is a particularly powerful, authoritative, legitimizing opportunity structure. In this case, teaching eugenics explicitly, or even simply asking students to record their own family trees and then mail these to the Eugenics Record Office (access Krisch), these curricular inclusions created the environment in which eugenics could germinate and grow as a movement.

In 1911, a leader of the American eugenics movement, Charles Davenport wrote the extremely influential *Heredity in Relation to Eugenics*, a book that "was assigned reading in many of the eugenics courses that were springing up at colleges and universities across the country, and was cited in more than one-third of the high school biology textbooks of the era" (Cohen, 112). In the book he suggested that "summarizing the review of recent conditions of immigration," after he had looked in depth at each group, "it appears certain that, unless conditions change of themselves or are radically changed, the population of the United States will, on account of the great influx of blood from South-Eastern Europe, rapidly become darker in pigmentation, smaller in stature, more mercurial, more attached to music and art, more given to crimes of larceny, kidnapping, assault, murder, rape, and sex-immorality" (219). This was the lesson being taught in North American classrooms.

We also know that the American Eugenics Society, for instance, began to reach out to American intellectuals to insinuate eugenic rhetoric into American higher education. As Henry Laughlin, one of the leaders of the Society wrote, in 1922:

Teachers of biology, sociology and psychology are finding it profitable to include in their practical laboratory work, provisions for building up, by the research method, authentic family histories with special reference to the descent and recombination of natural physical and mental qualities. . . . the average University student is able to compile a valuable biological record of the family within a few months' time. This record centers about the student himself, and, thus, when analyzed, throws light upon the origin of his natural capacities and limitations, and upon his potentiality as a parent in passing on particular traits. (3)

He continues: "this cooperative work promises to be not only profitable from the standpoint of the University giving the particular course, but also in building up biological family records of the better American families" (4). In 1925, 1,457 of these records were collected.

Angus McLaren argues that, for Canadian eugenicists, their final "chief success" was "in popularizing biological arguments" (67). And as

Francis Galton wrote in his 1909 *Chapters in Eugenics*, "The first and main point is to secure the general intellectual acceptance of Eugenics as a hopeful and most important study. Then let its principles work into the heart of the nation, who will gradually give practical effect to them in ways that we may not wholly foresee" (43). Clearly, getting eugenics into the curriculum of higher education was a way to plant a seed.

So, the actual curriculum at North American colleges and universities both fueled the rise of eugenics and allowed eugenics to continue to be taught in more subtle or covert ways well after the Holocaust. If you doubt this, I encourage you to search the historical course catalogues at your own school for the word eugenics.

Not only did eugenics actually reshape the North American population through things like immigration restriction, not only did it reshape families through its campaigns for "better breeding," not only did it reshape bodies through medical intervention, but it reshaped how North Americans thought about bodies and minds.

Academia is implicated very deeply in this history. Academia was the place from which eugenic "science" gained its funding and legitimization so that eugenicists could undertake massive projects in both "positive" and "negative" eugenics. But the university was also itself a laboratory for "positive" eugenics, a place where the "right" combinations of genes could be brought together ("the better families") and where eugenic ideals and values could be conveyed to the future teachers, lawyers, doctors, and other professionals on campus.

As Craig Steven Wilder showed in his landmark study of the racist roots of academia, *Ebony and Ivy*, in the United States, "European powers deployed colleges to help defend and regulate their colonial possessions and they turned to [the slave trade] to fund these efforts" (9). "College founders and officers used enslaved people to raise buildings, maintain campuses, and enhance their institutional wealth" while they also "trained the personnel and cultivated the ideas that accelerated and legitimated the dispossession of Native Americans and the enslavement of Africans" (Wilder, 10). Other U.S. college founders raised money from England, ostensibly to educate "barbarian" natives. Henry Dunster, Harvard's president, did so when his institution was running low on cash—building the Indian college in 1654 (Wright, 78). These founders raised money to convert "lost heathens" but really furthered "their own political, economic and educational agendas, which included Indian education as an ancillary aim at best" while they acted pious and righteous, while they "revitalized [their] colonial enterprises" (Wright, 78).

In Canada, with a different but similarly devastating history of enslavement and dispossession, (nonetheless) university founders relied on what Ian Mosby calls "colonial science." I would define that as experimentation on aboriginal peoples in the name of or under the disguise of reeducation or assimilation, as well as the depletion of their connections to the environment and the deletion of their own forms of knowledge. This colonial science was thoroughly institutionalized and reinforced by government policy, at the same time establishing the knowledge and power of universities. These eugenic practices, and in fact eugenics itself, can be seen as the invention of the North American university, which in turn was also built upon the exploitation of people with disabilities. Colleges and universities were colonial projects—places for settlers to continue the work of forcibly changing their landscapes and these landscapes' inhabitants, but also as sites of a sort of internalized imperialism, because universities were mainly where North Americans went to Europeanize. Eugenics was not just implicated in these moves, but was in many ways the perfect ideological vehicle for the settler colonialism of higher education. More simply, academia became the place where North Americans could most efficiently destroy what and who came before European settlement. Eugenics—the idea that certain bodies were biologically inferior—was rhetorical fuel for this very efficient destruction.

In Canada, there has been some public acknowledgment of this history, following the Canadian government's settlement and apology for the ongoing abuse of aboriginal children in residential schools. As the opening passage of the Canadian *Truth and Reconciliation Report*, developed as part of this ongoing apology, states: "For over a century, the central goals of Canada's Aboriginal policy were to eliminate Aboriginal governments; ignore Aboriginal rights; terminate the Treaties; and, through a process of assimilation, cause Aboriginal peoples to cease to exist as distinct legal, social, cultural, religious, and racial entities in Canada" (1). As indigenous scholar Richard Atleo writes in *Principles of Tsawalk*, the evolutionary ideas of Darwin were effectively transformed into eugenic rhetorics that were employed against indigenous people because they "created, for colonizers, a view of differences between people that was and is characterized by superiority and inferiority" (9). Absorbed early into political and imperialist domination ideologies, Darwin's theories of natural determinism justified the white European's central mythological conviction of racial superiority (Saul, 9). As Canadian public intellectual John Ralston Saul writes, "Canadians of

European origin decided that 'Indians,' 'Half-breeds' and 'Esquimaux' were among the destined losers when faced by our superiority—our Darwinian destiny" (12).

Immediately below, I am about to provide some specific evidence of this eugenic research, and it is potentially upsetting or triggering.

As Mosby and others have proven, universities provided the capital and the research to solidify this invented superiority. Mosby's research, for instance, reveals that children at residential schools were used in nutritional experiments. As further evidence continues to be uncovered, it is clear that these indigenous children were seen as readily available research resources. The construction of native youth as eugenically inferior coincided with their usage as test subjects. They were disabled by eugenic and settler colonial ideology and then disabled—literally, starved—by science.

As James W. Trent, author of *Inventing the Feeble Mind*, and others have shown, the history of eugenic research, testing, and promotion at Western institutions such as Stanford and Harvard shows us that universities have been the arbiter of ability and the inventor of disability as a sign of eugenic deterioration—as the evidence that somehow some genes, some racial groups, were innately disabled. North American academics have delineated and disciplined the border between able and disabled. These line-drawers were able to solidify their own positions as they closed the doors upon others. The disabled, in this history, were more than left out: disabled people have been experimented upon, sterilized, imprisoned, and killed.

As Trent has pointed out, North American academics systematically developed the means to segregate society based upon arbitrary ideas of ability—the university was the place for the most able, the mental institution or asylum or school for the "feeble-minded" the space for the "least." Charles Benedict Davenport, a Harvard PhD and instructor, and David Starr Jordan, president of Stanford University, are recognized as the fathers of the U.S. eugenics movement. Davenport, perhaps the eugenics movement's greatest proponent, defined the movement as "the science of the improvement of the human race by better breeding" (in Quigley, 1). The eugenics movement resulted in the institutionalization of millions of North Americans in asylums, "idiot schools," and other warehousing institutions, where people were abused, neglected, and, often, forcibly sterilized. Many children from large immigrant families were shipped to these "asylum schools," women were incarcerated as "hysterical," and they housed a radically disproportionate number of indigenous people, African Americans, Eastern Europeans, and lower-class children, all expendable according to eugenic thinking. Starr Jordan and Davenport worked to apply these ideas to bodies they deemed weak, and this was all made possible by the privileged position of these men within North America's "finest schools." These leaders didn't just make universities their own platforms for their own eugenic ideas; they made universities societal platforms for the very popular movement of eugenics; they made universities both places where you could learn about eugenics, and they created universities as experiments and laboratories for eugenics, built out of bricks and mortar.

As Heather Munro Prescott, a medical historian, has shown, "by the late 1920s, more than three hundred colleges and universities offered courses that covered eugenic themes, with as many as twenty thousand students enrolled" (102). Hygiene departments at these schools also advocated for "euthenics," "the notion that American racial stock in general could be improved through better nutrition, health care, and other preventive health measures" (102), and colleges and universities were some of the best places to implement these measures. Mental hygiene programs became prevalent at U.S. schools in the '20s and '30s. Despite this, many schools did not want to publicize their presence: "faculty members were skeptical of mental hygienists, believing them to be coddling students who could not meet standards" because "the popular conflation of mental illness and mental 'defectiveness' was all too common" (120, 121). These efforts proved to be tinged by homophobia and antisemitism, and powerfully shaped by sexism: "the focus on protecting women's bodies and minds reflected widely-held beliefs about the physical and mental characteristics of the "weaker sex"" while "concerns about race suicide and racial degeneration would surface in discussions about the health of college men, serving to justify the development of hygiene programs aimed at building their bodies along with their brains" (29). Thus "sex education programs, in the form of family life education, sought not only to control the spread of venereal disease but also to eradicate the 'homosexual menace' on campus" (127). It's not much of a leap to begin to understand how these two projects came at odds on "coeducational" campuses: How could women be protected while men were also encouraged to propagate? As Andrew Lucchesi shows, at many schools (including the City University of New York, where he traces a specific lineage) the mental hygiene or student health movements led directly into the creation of disability services offices. Elsewhere, or sometimes concurrently, these led to counseling offices and the current trend of "campus wellness," which might be defined as a kind of hybrid of mental hygiene and physical health.

Not only did eugenic ideas actually reshape the North American body, eugenics reshaped how North Americans thought about bodies and minds, and this had overt curricular reinforcement. But more than this, as Eileen Welsome, James Trent, Vera Hassner Sharav, and others have argued, institutional basements were labs for the social and biological experimentation of scholars from the Ivory Towers. For instance, institutions for "feeble minded" children like Wrentham or Fernald in Boston were tightly connected to Harvard and MIT. Wrentham was opened in 1906. In the 1950s, "residents" at this and the Fernald School (founded 1854) were fed radioactive isotopes in a scientific experiment. Young boys at these schools signed up to be part of the "science club," a name invented by the MIT faculty, and they were given Mickey Mouse watches and armbands, and taken on special outings, in return for taking part in a "nutritional study." Seventy-four boys were fed oatmeal injected with radioactive iron or calcium (Welsome, 231, 235). Welsome suggests there was "nothing unique" about this study, as the school had become a "veritable laboratory" with a "captive population" for academics from Boston (231, 233).

I could go on: Paul Yakovlev, a Harvard scientist and resident doctor at several institutions, built a collection of nearly 1,000 brains, turning institution morgues into labs and making some young boys dissect these specimens (Welsome, 233). His collection was later donated to Harvard, where they are still proudly displayed. Fernald School came to be known by Boston academics as "the zoo" because of the wide range of ailments represented there, and the bodies held there for easy viewing and study. Many of the pictures used (and still found) in medical textbooks came from these schools. These phrenological and physiognomical (now renamed "neuropathological") studies, along with the genetic studies of eugenicist like Henry Goddard and others at such institutions, led to a catalogue of dysgenic deterioration, the inverse of the pursuit of perfection at the university. Upward academic movement was fueled by the objectified bodies and minds in these basements, which the steep steps also reached down towards.

Let's remember as well the fact that this entire map of academia is already superimposed over indigenous land that was stolen, swindled, appropriated. For instance, when Harvard created their aforementioned Indian College in the 1650s, they did so by grabbing a parcel of land that had not long ago been forcibly taken from the Wampanoag—so that they could turn around and Christianize the Wampanoag, most of whom became terribly sick from attending Harvard, while others were killed as traitors for working as research assistants to Harvard professors like John Eliot (access Blood and Land by J. C. H King). On the campus of my undergraduate alma mater, the University of British Columbia, a longhouse was built on campus with the collaboration of the local Musqueam First Nation, and opened around the time that I was a student there. What wasn't included? The surrounding nearly 1,000 acres of land that had, since time immemorial, been an educational ground for the Musqueam, and continues to be the traditional, ancestral, unceded territory of the Musqueam people. UBC has now fully monetized all of this land—converting this Musqueam territory first by building campus buildings and housing, but then by creating a UBC Real Estate Corporation to develop condominiums, condos that now sell, at a minimum, for $1.5 million, bringing 8,000 private residents onto campus in under 30 years, and growing the university's endowment from $100 million to $1.2 billion as a result (access Rosenfeld). Campus mapping decidedly cannot begin just when the first academic building goes up. And clearly, one entailment of colonial development is that all available resources will be extracted as efficiently as possible.

In Canada, since their very beginnings, universities were deeply invested in making careful, long-term investments in social and even agricultural programs to erase First Nations (access Daschuk). Even more specifically, "during the war and early postwar period—bureaucrats, doctors, and scientists recognized the problems of hunger and malnutrition, yet increasingly came to view Aboriginal bodies as 'experimental materials' and residential schools and Aboriginal communities as kinds of 'laboratories' that they could use to pursue a number of different political and professional interests" (Mosby, 148). The scientists' ambitions were always more powerful and clear than their ethics. "In the end, these studies did little to alter the structural conditions that led to malnutrition and hunger in the first place and, as a result, did more to bolster the career ambitions of the researchers than to improve the health of those identified as being malnourished" (Mosby, 148). Further, "the early architects of Canada's residential school system saw the schools as social laboratories in which people's beliefs and ways could be refashioned. But as these experiments made clear, the systematic neglect and mistreatment of students in these schools also made them into ideal scientific laboratories" (Mosby, 162). What has not been studied as deeply—or, really, at all—in Canada is that such experiments have also been performed on people with disabilities for over one hundred years. For instance, the Children's Psychiatric Research Institute, a residential "school" in London, Ontario, was in part established because researchers from the University of Western Ontario were tired of having to travel all the way to Orillia, Ontario, to access patients and research subjects at the Hospital School there (access Zarfas). This research strengthened the career ambitions of the researchers, and the research reputations of the universities from which they came.

Institutions like the Hospital School also benefited greatly from their affiliation with research and academia. As Julia Oparah similarly shows, collaborations with universities have provided corporations, government initiatives, and the industrial complex in the United States with technology and with research capital, but also with "moral capital because of their association with progressive values" and "liberal credentials" (101).[2] Universities have generally been given a blank check and open doors to perform research at North American spaces of incarceration for over a 150 years, and in so doing have fortified these exclusionary spaces and strengthened them by wrapping them in academic values. Bringing in academics to head asylums and "idiot schools" brought moral capital as well; association with universities likely protected these segregated spaces from more careful public scrutiny and critique.

Thus, one way to map the spaces of academia and disability would be to look at the ways land was parceled out in North America in the late 1800s (parceling that always took place as though this was settlers' land to divide up as they pleased). While universities were popping up in urban settings and on land grant tracts, asylums and "idiot schools" were popping up in other, nearby rural settings—on old farms and "abandoned" land. Yet the two institutions were often tightly hinged or yoked together. For instance, as Katie Aubrecht has shown, the University of Toronto had roots as an asylum for women (9). Later, the same buildings expanded, multiplied, and the university became a colonial "experiment" as a place to reproduce British traditions on stolen land (9).

From within one privileged space, academics were deciding the fate of others in similar (sometimes identical), yet somehow now pathological, other, and impure spaces. This eugenic program relied on the attribution of disability to society's Others and is tightly connected to scientific racism and sexism, compulsory heterosexuality, the control of reproductive rights, the creation a bifurcated workforce, even a global capitalist system. The legacy of this invention is still part of our academic identity.

Snapshots of Exclusion

In these ways, disability has been studied at the university and at the college, where research has also advanced a series of disabling studies. Yet this book is featured within one of the first book series in North America devoted to disability studies as an academic discipline. Thus you might think that there will be a narrative of progress here, moving toward more equitable approaches to disability and a disavowal of the legacy of academic eugenics.

Yet as disability studies scholar David Bolt and others have shown, even though "disability is relevant to most if not all disciplines" in the contemporary academy, there is a "critical avoidance [and a] lack of critical engagement" with disability that evidences a "manifestly academic form of Othering" (2). While academics will talk about health, or the body, they will rarely talk about disability studies, rarely engage with the authority of disabled people on these matters, and rarely locate their work within the field of disability studies itself. As David Mitchell argues, the root cause of this is "unabashed commitment of universities to the reproduction of practitioners of normalization as the terms of exchange in the awarding of higher education degrees" (18–19). Universities create doctors and special educators and therapists who learn how to rehabilitate or cure disability, or how to tokenize or minimally include it. Seeing disability as fixable is very, very different from seeing disability as desirable, or understanding disability subjectivity as diversifying a "stagnating cultural knowledge base about differential embodiment" (David Mitchell, 19). In short, educating people to erase and diminish disability ensures limitations on our knowledge about bodies and minds.

Moreover, the continued struggle to fight for small accommodations for students with disabilities also ensures that perhaps we are now in the era of people with disabilities fighting to get the chance to study at all. Educators must recognize both the long history of exclusion and experimentation upon people with disabilities, as well as the more recent history of academic ableism experienced by disabled students. I begin this exploration with some numbers, and some anecdotal facts, all wrapped together to give a snapshot of disability and higher education today.

The university sorts the population by a medicalized and legalistic definition of "ability" as effectively now as it ever has. Universities continue to function to keep certain groups of individuals out of the work force and away from status positions, and away from knowledge and dialogue and power, and not just through admissions. Thirteen percent of U.S. citizens 25 and older with a disability have a bachelor's degree or higher. This compares with 31 percent for those with no disability (Census). Twenty-seven percent of Canadians have university degrees. But only 17.6 percent of Canadians with "mild or moderate" disabilities have postsecondary degrees, and only 8.8 percent of those with "severe or very severe" disabilities have a degree (Statistics Canada). In the United Kingdom, "disabled people are around 3 times as likely not to hold any qualifications compared to non-disabled people, and around half as likely to hold a degree-level qualification" (UK Labour).

While, recently, more students with disabilities are enrolling than in previous eras in the United States, "nearly two thirds are unable to complete their degrees within six years" (Smith, n.p.). This shows how the university is a sorting gate but also a holding pen. This impact is doubled for students with disabilities because if they do graduate it takes them at least 25 percent longer to complete the same degree requirements as non-disabled students (Looker and Lowe). Just 41 percent of students with learning disabilities complete their postsecondary education, compared to 52 percent of the U.S. general population (Cortiella and Horowitz; Walpole and Chaskes). As Wessel et al. show, "students with disabilities, when compared with their counterparts without disabilities, were more likely to delay their college attendance a year or more after finishing high school (43 versus 32 percent). They were also more likely to have earned a GED or alternative high school credential (12 versus 6 percent), to have dependents other than a spouse (25 versus 13 percent), and to have financial and family obligations that potentially conflicted with their schooling" (117).

Disabled students are likely to have up to 60 percent more student debt by the time they graduate.[3] As Sarah Mohamed reveals, "debt is particularly onerous for students with disabilities who consequently require more time to complete their degree or diploma [and] this is a major contributing factor to persons with disabilities having lower application, admission and graduation rates as well as higher rates of leaving and switching programs" (n.p.). These statistics are skewed because they only account for the students who receive accommodations. What would the overall retention and graduation rates be for all students with disabilities regardless of documentation or accommodation? Because despite the fact that one in seven Canadians has a disability, only 2 percent of Canadian students actually seek disability accommodations and—unbelievably—8 percent of Canadian colleges or universities have reported having no students with disabilities at all (Fichten et al.). The simple extrapolation tells us that at least 100,000 and probably more like 200,000 Canadian postsecondary students need accommodations but never seek them. In the United States, some studies show that two-thirds of college students "don't receive accommodations simply because their colleges don't know about their disabilities" (Grasgreen, n.p.). Those who do seek accommodations are likely to do so only in their third or fourth year of school. In the UK, in 2015/2016, 176,480 postsecondary students were known to have a disability—that's 12.29 percent (Higher Education Statistical Agency). According to the most recent statistics, published in 2016, in the United States, 11.1 percent students were known to have disabilities (National Center for Education Statistics). But whatever the numbers, and whatever the statistics tell us about how dire prospects might be for disabled students, the statistics only speak for the very small number of disabled students who successfully navigate the complicated accommodation process to seek help.

The economics of accommodation might tell us that universities get the outcomes they pay for. The most recent Association of Higher Education and Disability (2008) survey of U.S. disability services offices revealed that "the average annual DS office budget was $257,289 (SD=$306,471)" (Harbour, 41). The numbers in Canada are very similar. That's the entire office budget. That is about what a dean at an Ontario university makes, on average. It's about what any U.S. college pays its chancellor. It's less than one-sixth of the average salary for a U.S. college football coach. So a dean or assistant coach makes as much in a year as the average school spends on all students with disabilities. Deans and football coaches are also seeing their salaries climb precipitously. Those are growth industries. The same can't be said for these office budgets. The ratio at these offices was one staff member per 80 students with disabilities (Harbour, 52). In Canada, there are barely more than 200 professionals employed to provide disability accommodations at Canadian colleges and universities, and so the rough staff-to-student ratio or "caseload" is somewhere between 1:125 to 1:250 (Fichten et al., 73).[4] Offices of disability services are thus clearly overworked and underfunded. Thus we shouldn't really be surprised that the number of college and university students identified as having disabilities is drastically below the average within the general population. It shouldn't be surprising that, for instance, while 94 percent of learning-disabled high school students get assistance, only 17 percent of college students with learning disabilities do (Krupnick, n.p.).[5] These offices are already working above capacity, and may have implicit incentives or restraints, or both, that minimize the supports they can offer and the ways that students might be able to access assistance. This underfunding also tells the rest of the university that disability doesn't matter.

The underfunding should also be linked to other pressing trends in higher education. For instance, the impact on disabled faculty is similarly remarkable. As a teacher using the pseudonym Alice K. Adjunct wrote in a *Disability Studies Quarterly* article in 2008:

> Unfortunately, the opportunities for Ph.D.s with disabilities to become full professors are growing less, rather than more, available. Research suggests that there is still a pervasive atmosphere of malignant neglect toward faculty accommodation. This neglect, coupled with the explosively expanding shift toward an adjunct, rather than tenured, academic workforce bode ill for aspiring professors with disabilities. The adjunct economy adds yet one more inherent workplace disadvantage to the load of them already borne . . . by new Ph.D.s with disabilities. (n.p.)

Recent statistics show very low numbers of tenure-track professors with disabilities nationwide: just 3.6 percent, based on a U.S. Department of Education study in 2004. There is no data available on the exact number of disabled professors pushed into the adjunct ranks, but given the general trends around employment discrimination against disabled people, we can assume that the majority of disabled Ph.D.s who do teach, do so as adjuncts. As Alice K. Adjunct wrote, "meanwhile, students suffer. The low pay, negligible administrative support and packed schedules inherent to the adjunct system prevent able-bodied professors from doing their best for their students" and "these barriers to great teaching loom even higher for adjunct lecturers with disabilities" (n.p.).[6]

On the other side of the scale of academic prestige and privilege, the managerial class on campuses has grown. And since the 2008 financial crisis, student debt has risen precipitously. What's the connection? Interestingly, the universities in the United States with the top 25 highest executive pay rates also had the worst student debt crisis, with "the sharpest rise in student debt . . . when executive compensation soared the highest"; with "administrative spending outstripping scholarship spending by more than 2 to 1 at state schools with the highest-paid presidents"; with "part-time adjunct faculty increasing 22 percent faster than the national average" at these schools while "permanent faculty declined dramatically as a percentage of all faculty" (Wood and Erwin, n.p.). All of these statistics come from Marjorie Wood and Andrew Erwin's study "The One Percent at State U," in which they suggest that "state universities have come under increasing criticism for excessive executive pay, soaring student debt, and low-wage faculty labor. In the public debate, these issues are often treated separately," but their "findings suggest these issues are closely related and should be addressed together in the future" (n.p.). While I am unable to connect their data with rates of investment in disability services and with the adjunctification of disabled PhDs, it is certain that the drop in scholarship money and the general increase in student debt impacts disabled students disproportionately, and that the rise of the academic "one percent" is bad for all students— and most teachers, amplifying the employment discrimination that disabled people experience.

But the structural and financial details are just one part of this picture because the process of seeking accommodations for those students who actually do try to do access them is so difficult, the path strewn with barriers.

Students with disabilities often meet peers who have little familiarity with disabilities, hold stigmas about people with disabilities, or even consider academic accommodations for students with disabilities to be an unfair advantage (Olney & Kim). It is not uncommon for students with disabilities to find themselves in a position of explaining to faculty details about eligibility for accommodations, the accommodation process, and the range of available support to students with disabilities on campus (Cawthon & Cole; Ryan). These same faculty are very likely to believe— just as students do—that the accommodations are an unfair advantage (O'Shea and Meyer).

For most students who seek accommodations for our classes, they aren't allowed to know what the actual range of accommodations might be. Instead, they have to go in to disability services, offer up their diagnosis, and have that diagnosis matched with a stock set of accommodations. In other exchanges, students might be asked by disability services to "tell us what you need"—and again students have to guess. Just imagine how much further this disadvantages students from other cultures, first-generation college and university students, and other students who might not fully understand the culture of higher education. Throughout the book, I will explore the toll this accommodation process takes.

Another crucial but drastically understudied aspect of disability in higher education: How does disability diagnosis intersect with other markers of difference? We know that "African American males are disproportionately placed into categories of special education that are associated with extremely poor outcomes" at the K-12 level (Losen and Gillespie). Yet education researcher Joy Banks has shown that "African American students with disabilities experience difficulty accessing disability support services and appropriate accommodations" at colleges and universities (28). So how can it be that for the same group of students, a disability diagnosis at the K-12 level can be hastily applied, and will speed them into the school-to-prison pipeline, and at the postsecondary level is so much more difficult to get? As Michelle Alexander, author of *The New Jim Crow*, points out in an interview:

> [Y]outh of color, particularly those in ghetto communities, find themselves born into the cage. . . . The cage is the unequal educational opportunities these children are provided at a very early age coupled with the constant police surveillance they're likely to encounter, making it very likely that they're going to serve time. Middle-class white children, children of privilege, are afforded the opportunity to make a lot of mistakes and still go on to college, still dream big dreams. But for kids who are born in the ghetto in the era of mass incarceration, the system is designed in such a way that it traps them, often for life." (n.p.)

Further bars within this cage metaphor, then, are the disability diagnoses that might be applied to these students.

What about international students? While many schools are targeting these students and charging them quite a bit more tuition than domestic students, and while the number of international students in the West climbs every year, very few schools consider the difficulty these students may have getting the diagnoses required to obtain accommodations, or dealing with other linguistic and cultural barriers to access.[7] Will they be eligible for government support programs? How will they access doctors? Will diagnostic tests even be offered in languages other than English? Is the passive approach to their support in fact a form of immigration restriction? That is, if higher education is a pathway to recruiting talented immigrants, could a lack of disability support act to filter out disabled immigrants?

As Marjorie Johnstone and Eunjung Lee point out,

> currently, the world's primary education hosts are the colonizing countries and the offshoot white settler societies from the 19th-century age of imperialism. . . . This exchange contributes to Western nation-building and reduces the capacity of source countries to build their own knowledge economy with research and education based on their own resources and power. In a marriage with neoliberal ideas, this exchange decimates national social welfare systems, thus increasing wealth disparities, inequality, and the oppression of marginalized populations (such as newcomers, racialized, disabled and gendered groups) while fostering private purchase of social services (e.g. education brokers, tutoring, and counseling). (219)

In short, international education can be disabling on a global scale. As Patricia McLean, Margaret Heagney, and Kay Gardner argue, "as global educational opportunities expand, the implications for students with a disability must also be considered; not to do so is potentially discriminatory" (226). Though statistics were unavailable in North America, Higher Education Strategy Associates show that "between 2001/02 to 2004/05, the percentage increase in disabled international students entering British higher education (38.24 per cent) exceeds both disabled domestic students (37.02 per cent) and non-disabled international students (31.38 per cent)" (quoted in Soorenian, n.p.).

I offer this tangle of citations, this stack of numbers not as decisive facts—the numbers shift, and they are used from a wide variety of angles to make a wide variety of arguments. Someone might use many of the same numbers or studies I have tangled up here to fashion a strong warning about the ways students with disabilities are infiltrating higher education, for instance, or to encourage teachers and administrators to panic, or to argue for exclusive programs.

It may seem that we have moved through the approach, mentioned at the beginning of this book, away from the era of eugenics, and toward an era of access, fueled by the disability rights movement and the rise of academic disability studies. But a few facts are irrefutable. Students with disabilities are still kept out of the university in large numbers. Disabled students will face steep steps as they work to attain an education. The programs and initiatives that are developed in the name of diversity and inclusion do not yet deliver tangible means of addressing the ableism inherent in higher education.

In Wendy Brown's *Undoing the Demos*, a powerful critique of the concept of diversity as it has been evoked in higher education, she identifies three eras in academic history in North America.

1. First a focus on "developing intelligent thoughtful elites and reproducing culture";
2. Then a focus on "enacting a principle of equal opportunity and cultivating a broadly educated citizenry";
3. Now, higher education "produces human capital, thereby turning classically humanist values on their head." (Brown, 24)

In Brown's scheme, the first step unequivocally, undoubtedly excluded disability, and folded the invention of disability into the mission of those inside elites. This was the eugenics era, and academics were very actively involved in this work, and founded universities on eugenic research. As I mentioned at the beginning of this introduction: disability has always been constructed as the inverse or opposite of higher education. Or, as I put it more simply: higher education has needed to create a series of versions of "lower education" to justify its work and to ground its exceptionalism. This was the era of disabling studies and disability studied.

The second step—the use of higher education as a principle of equal opportunity—opened many doors and removed many barriers, but all too often disability was used to test the edges of opportunity; for people with disabilities, the equal access promised by the second step never really came, or only ever came in a qualified way. Here, while the discourse or discussion about disability was about welcoming and including, the back end was being built to construct disability purely under what might be called a medical and a liability model: define disability medically, treat it in a legalistic, minimalistic manner designed to avoid getting sued. This can force accommodation to happen, but it also tends to force—always and only—the legal minimum accommodation. Disabled people, then, come to have their experiences of education shaped by these legal minimums. That's a difficult way to learn, and a difficult way to live.

Now the concept of equality has been co-opted by the third step, wherein disability, like other forms of embodied difference, gets commodified. As Zahari Richter powerfully writes, "ableist knowledge production consists of the knowledge practices of constituting disabled people entirely through detached observation and disembodied gazing or studying practices" (n.p.). Disabled people are objects for education, not subjects or agents of it. In this scheme, disability might be mentioned as a unique "special" part of the fabric of society, universities and colleges might preach inclusiveness and promote neoliberal values like diversity, but in the end disability is still just studied, and the impact continues to be disabling in the sense of further distancing disability from power and further stigmatizing disability.

In this book, I will study all three of these "eras" of disability in higher education, matching these eras with spatial metaphors and mapping them across specific disciplines within the university. Yet *Academic Ableism* is written from the third era, the era in which students and teachers find themselves today, within the neoliberal university.

It is "neoliberalism" that Wendy Brown is defining in *Undoing the Demos* when she suggests that humanist values have been overtaken by a focus on human capital—or the economic value that might be gained or taken from human bodies and their work. Liberal values then become the things that economic motivations hide behind. Cash rules everything around modern higher education, and cash rules most effectively when it can be hidden behind values like individual choice and responsibility. More simply, higher education is an industry which, beyond the surface, is dominated by economic considerations, but most of the time doesn't want to be seen as a business. Perhaps more dangerously, because higher education does champion values like autonomy, freedom of expression, and creativity, it becomes altogether too easy to ignore its economic character. Unsurprisingly, but also depressingly, higher education is a neoliberal business like any other. Maybe this is because governments have been cutting funding to schools, maybe it is because the managerial class within universities knows no other way. Regardless, unlike other businesses, higher education is highly capable of disguising the dominance of economic considerations behind liberal values.

The result is that the rich—rich students, rich administrators, rich institutions—get richer. Those who need higher education to "get ahead" don't have the same path to success as those who are already privileged. As Mark Bousquet argues, workers in education "have seen the compulsory acceleration of market behavior (such as competition for resources and profit-seeking) in their professional cultures. . . . the management of professional activities has resulted in the return of . . . dizzying inequalities" (1). In his words: "If it sounds a bit Orwellian, or a bit like Foucault goes to business school, it should" (12). Henry Giroux also argues that we need to "connect the dots between the degradation of higher education and those larger economic, political, cultural and social forces that benefit from" this degradation (129). Neoliberalism is more than a "set of economic policies," it is a "normative order of reason developed over three decades into a widely and deeply disseminated governing rationality [that] transmogrifies every human domain and endeavor, along with humans themselves, according to a specific image of the economic. All conduct is economic conduct" (Brown, 10). Universities, colleges, and the industries that orbit them benefit from this conduct while the vast majority of students do not. This understanding of imbalanced benefit and harm, then, must be used to examine the workings of academic ableism.

Who benefits in academia, today, from the inclusions and exclusions of disabled students, and who hides these inclusions and exclusions behind other liberal values? For instance, and as a means to avoid creating a narrative of progress for disability in higher education, what is the likely future "economic conduct" of ableism and disability? Who seems to be investing, who is benefiting from, and who is paying the costs for ableism? Well, online courses are growing at a rate of 10 times the growth of on-site classes, and more than 20 percent of U.S. students took an online course in fall 2007 (Allen and Seaman). That jumped to 33.5 percent in 2013 (Allen and Seaman). How can we ensure that these courses are going to be accessible to all students? How will we guard against an impulse that is the seeming inverse of this inaccessibility? That is, how will we make sure that students with disabilities are not going to be funneled away from on-site classes and into online classes as a method of exclusion?

What about at the level of admissions? As Jennifer Doyle points out, the "administration wants students who are richer and better educated. How do we get better students? How do we get students who need less from us?" (97). Yet other colleges recognize disabled students as a particularly promising market. Segregated colleges now exist for students with learning disabilities, and, within regular colleges, many extra support programs for students now also come with huge price tags. If some doors are opening wider, what other doors are closing? If schools are providing minimal accommodations, and anything extra costs a lot, how are our colleges really responding to the diversity of learners?

There is also huge growth in programs like "disability management" at the same time that disability studies programs are in a holding pattern on most college campuses. Learning how to minimize and manage disability's impact on the workplace is an academic field that will likely continue to grow. Soon enough, unfortunately, the skills these students learn in minimizing and managing disability might make them ideal candidates to work on college campuses in disability resource offices. What does it mean that more and more students are learning that disability should be understood mainly as having a negative economic impact, one that needs to be creatively diminished?

Further, the growth of programs like "disability management" are generally aimed at a "relatively more homogenous population among the ranks of already-employed professionals and upper-level service workers," as Evan Watkins points out (Class, 93). These programs allow universities to grow without expanding undergraduate education. The expansion is tremendously efficient, as these professional programs usually charge premium tuition and draw very few students from "historically underserved student populations" (Class, 93). Combine this with the aspirations among elite schools towards what Sheila Slaughter and Larry L. Leslie call "academic capitalism": the entrepreneurial goals that place upper-level research and graduate programs above all else. This entrepreneurial research is highly likely to focus on curative approaches to disability and very unlikely to focus on disability as a rights or an identity issue. Thus academia begins to shape itself and brand itself through white-collar programs and enrollments, through curative research, as a way to expand financially without expanding access at the undergraduate level.

The huge industry of for-profit colleges like Everest and Phoenix also spend a disproportionate amount of their government funding on recruiting. Their recruiters are trained to exploit and "poke" the pain and sense of vulnerability and inadequacy of potential recruits (Kirkham). This poking of vulnerability was to have been a key issue in Donald Trump's Trump University fraud trial (it was settled out of court for $25 million). As the business of these colleges grows, they will certainly find new ways to exploit disabled students for the government grants that might be attached to their enrollment.

An expanded understanding of a wider range of disabilities has also led to a rhetorical outpouring of troubling language: students with emotional and psychological disabilities are characterized according to their "warning signs" (Erdur-Baker et al.); students with PTSD are seen to be "ticking time bombs" and more segregated programs are being created for veterans within U.S. colleges; autism is seen as a costly "epidemic" that is now hitting higher education (Cowen, n.p.). How to we respond to this stigmatization? How can we recognize the eugenic undercurrent in such discourse?

Each of these new developments may translate into a different future—an opportunity to shape or be shaped according to the diversity of the students in the classroom. The goal, then, is to create an approach that recognizes the long history of disability and higher education inflected by the current, often camouflaged, vectors of academic ableism, without separating eras or introducing neat progressions.

Of course, when we talk about the university, we are actually talking about just one relatively powerful example of a social structure. One can likely find similarities in the courthouse, the hospital, in K-12 education, public transportation, many modern workplaces and most old ones, and so on. So, I urge you to make these comparisons. Look for these steep steps and gates everywhere. Similarly, this book cannot diagnose all of the problems with the contemporary university, or dig deeply into the philosophies upon which universities are founded—at least not in great detail. But others can and should take this work further. What is it about the history or the philosophical foundations, or the map or the architecture, or the current mission or set of budgetary priorities of your own school that makes it particularly ableist, or more accommodating, or that allows the ineffectiveness of these accommodations to be obscured or hidden, or that leads to celebrations of inclusion and diversity that don't ring true or effect change?

Michel Foucault has a particularly powerful quote he used to defend his work against claims it was nihilistic, too negative: "power is everywhere, not that it engulfs everything, but that it comes from everywhere" (Sexuality, 122). Likewise, it is worth remembering that at the contemporary college or university, ableism is everywhere: not that it overwhelms all of the good schooling can do, not that it invalidates your teaching or your research, but that we are all responsible for looking for it, recognizing our roles in its circulation, and seeking change.

A Note on (Plain) Language and (Open) Access

In a *New Yorker* article, Joshua Rothman wrote that:

> Since the liberal-arts job market peaked, in the mid-seventies, the audience for academic work has been shrinking. Increasingly, to build a successful academic career you must serially impress very small groups of people (departmental colleagues, journal and book editors, tenure committees). . . . they have no choice but to aim for

very small targets. Writing a first book, you may have in mind particular professors on a tenure committee; miss that mark and you may not have a job. (n.p.)

This invention of an academic tone certainly felt like the process of writing my first book *Disability Rhetoric*—a book that has been praised by some for its accessibility and yet criticized by others for its use of academic jargon. I was so obsessed with worry about getting the work published that I was thinking about only a very small group of possible readers and reviewers. But the danger for a junior scholar is that we inflate our work with theory and with difficult language in an effort to sound as smart as possible. For disability studies researchers, this can mean that our work actually excludes members of our own community.

I would suggest that students and teachers of disability studies can add another dimension to the argument Joshua Rothman is making in the *New Yorker*, and argue that the process of making academic writing more and more academic can be a process of ableism and it can reproduce ableism, creating steep steps. Putting academic research in these terms matters.

One of the originators of disability studies, Tom Shakespeare wrote many years ago that "academic work on disability may not always be accessible. I believe writers should use plain language, but this does not equal a duty to be immediately comprehensible. I have quoted Einstein, who said 'Make everything as simple as possible. But not simpler'" (115). Jan Walmsley has similarly shown that "in learning disability research this debate [about plain language] is not aired. As far as inclusive research in learning disability goes, accessibility is central" because in this field plain language has always been incorporated (205). But Walmsley admits that her worry "is that inclusive researchers are so fearful of saying things which people with learning difficulties cannot follow that they say very little, leaving the field of theorising to others . . . with little or no commitment to inclusion" (205). My hope is that disability studies as a field will not follow this clear bifurcation or division between accessible and responsive researchers and inaccessible theorists. On these pages there will be an effort to create accessible theory, answerable to all. When it feels as though I am slipping into jargon or theory, I will stop and offer a simpler version. Often, the simpler version will also be the much better one. Sometimes, I will fail—that is the rhetorical nature of language, as something that relies upon context and audience to make meaning. But I will always make an effort to be plainly understood.

As Elizabeth Grace, an expert on disability and education, argues in a hugely influential article on the ways disability studies authors need to keep their work accessible, "in terms of access and justice, using plain language is very important. It's needed to allow the widest variety of people with disabilities to participate in conversations about themselves" (n.p.). Grace shows that this is an issue of economic justice as well. Yet, too often, writing in plain language "marks you as an outsider" and thus makes it difficult to access work, merit, and promotion, and "that's part of why we do not see it happen more often in certain fields of academic activity" (n.p.). Hopefully, my approach to plain language in this book—through the effort to both keep the prose relatively simple and to provide plain language summaries as often as possible—empowers others to similarly claim this outsider position. In so doing I hope it is possible to collapse some of the dynamics—the steep steps—that create an inside and an outside to begin with.[8]

In this same spirit, then, the book will be offered in an open access format. The book will be entirely free and offered in easily accessible digital format. The cost of academic publishing is a huge barrier that creates steep steps and ornate gates; insiders and outsiders. Further, print formats are difficult to access for many readers with disabilities. Making the book available for free in a digital format matters, and publishing the book in any other format would invalidate so many of its arguments.

The (now canonical) Bethesda Statement on the issue suggests that open access means anyone can access research on the public internet, for free, and "copy, use, distribute, transmit and display the work publicly and to make and distribute derivative works, in any digital medium for any responsible purpose, subject to proper attribution of authorship" (Suber et al., n.p.). Open access also centers the philosophy of the human "right to know" and "right to be known" (Willinsky, 7). That is, open access is a way of formatting and copyrighting scholarship, but it is also a philosophy: that information should be free and that if one hopes to actually engage with ideas (and to have them engaged with by others), rather than simply recording them on paper, the work needs to be made accessible.

That said, as Elizabeth Brewer, Melanie Yergeau, and Cynthia Selfe argue, "We have not, as yet, taken on the professional responsibility of making sure that all . . . [texts] are easily readable. . . . this is also true, of course, of many digital texts" (151). The truth is that in the push for open access, too much of the accessibility that comes along with it is just by chance and not by design—making it free is already half the battle, but it is also barely half the battle. So, in this spirit, this book will be offered in an open access and accessible format.

To have an accessible dissemination or movement of research, the reception and reading of texts needs to be considered in terms of accessibility—this expands the author's responsibility. But the means of distribution and reproduction also need to be reconsidered in terms of accessibility. You're printing a book? How much does it cost and how easy is it to read, for all possible readers? How freely do our ideas really move, and how difficult is it for some to access them and use them? Which bodies can take up texts and move (with) them? How does research get to those who have been excluded from the academy? If we understand rhetoric as the circulation of power and discourse through the body, then we need to ask how some of the "products" of academia do and do not move or circulate through a wide range of possible bodies.[9] How could this conversation move through the widest range of possible bodies?

Lessons about inclusion and exclusion extend from the physical spaces of the university, to its virtual spaces and movements. When we think about access, we also need to understand that most of the scholarly conversation in academia is not at all accessible. Further, most of the web is not at all accessible. Just as one means of illustrating this, in 2007, Thompson et al., using fairly robust criteria, tested a huge sample of government and education websites from hundreds of countries, internationally, to try and assess their accessibility. In the United States, only 45 percent of these pages even used text equivalents to describe visual elements and images, only 50 percent followed HTML standards, and only 24 percent "passed" basic navigational criteria.[10] The research is a bit old now—but the fact that there is very little knowledge or proactive action about what is a huge problem, disenfranchising such a huge segment of the world population, speaks to how little most people ever think about accessibility, believing instead that the web is generally open and free and that is all that matters.

As just one example of this accessibility, the images in this book will be fully and carefully described and given alt text in their digital format. Too often, books and articles skip adding in these additional descriptions, making the images, charts, graphs, and figures that may be central to their argument inaccessible to many members of their audience. In fact, in this book, sometimes all I will offer is a thick visual description of an image, as a means of highlighting the rhetorical and translational value of doing this describing.

Coda: Ableist Apologia

To end this introduction, I want to directly address a response that the book might well receive from many readers: for some reading right now, it may seem as though of course higher education is ableist. This could come in the form of a conscious response, or an unconscious feeling. Of course higher education is ableist.

In response, I want to argue that academic ableism faces specific forces of disguise and submersion. Because the sentiment that of course higher education is ableist is rarely coupled with a concern about this state of our institutions, and it is the job of this book to show how this ableism is a problem, and what can be done. But within academia, this feeling that there can be nothing done about the ableism of education, and that perhaps it is not even a problem, needs to be interrogated. What I would call "ableist apologia" describes a genre or category of statements and sentiments that distance the speaker from responsibility for the selective, stratifying forces within higher education, selecting and stratifying functions that depend upon ableism and disablism to make sure that privilege is portioned out only along traditional lines: to ensure that students who move, think, or express themselves outside of a narrow set of norms will not thrive or survive in college.

Apologia is a specific genre and has been understood by rhetoricians—as far back as Aristotle and likely much earlier than that—as speeches given in defense. Apologia are also, notably, connected to statements of regret. This description of an "affect" or emotion for apologia is particularly appropriate, as ableist apologies are often tinged with a sense of regret or fatigue, with the feeling that the apologizer is throwing their hands up in the air and saying: there's nothing I can do. Or a feeling that this is the last thing the apologizer is willing to do—that they are asked to do so much, that they do so much, and now they are also being asked to do more, to be more diligent. Other times, the apology comes simply in the form of: I didn't know. I'm sorry, I didn't know I was being ableist; I didn't know that was ableist. This claim of not-knowing is also, in a way, a claim that the ableism isn't really happening, isn't the case. This claim of not-knowing is also a claim to being a good person: separating the action or the implication from the individual. Because ableist apologia, as well, are rarely personal apologies—they are apologies for a state of affairs, not claims of individual responsibility. Too often, then, the emotion is not necessarily sincere and the apology is not exactly an apology at all.

Often, in the end, the apologies defend the apologizer and attempt to explain away their actions or inactions.

Ableist apologia happen when people say: yes, this building is inaccessible, but it's an old building (access Titchkosky, Question). Professors might say that a building is old as though they don't actively, currently teach and have an office with their name on it in that building. That one inhabits and uses a building every day means the building is alive. If it is an inaccessible building, it is alive and working to physically filter students out of the university every single day. It's not solely an old building, it's a living thing doing ableist work, and actively ignoring this allows it to do that work incredibly efficiently. Likewise, teachers apologize for ableism and refusals to accommodate by saying things like "I need to impose standards" or "I am preparing students for future classes" or even "I would be doing them a disservice if I didn't prepare them for what will come." But if stakeholders refuse to interrogate how these standards privilege particular bodies and minds, they help ableism disguise itself; they disguise it to themselves and to their students.

Yes, academia is ableist. In 1779, Thomas Jefferson proposed a two-track educational system, with different tracks, in his words, for "the laboring and the learned" (in Tyack, 89). Scholarships would allow a very few of the laboring class to advance, Jefferson said, by "raking a few geniuses from the rubbish" (in Tyack, 89). We could visit other sources to find the roots of higher education, and their sentiments might be similarly ableist or discriminatory. But this ableist reality is not something educators are committed to reproducing, doomed to repeat.

Another angle of this apologia is the idea that, if indeed academia is ableist, then everyone involved in education is, also. While this may be true, this is not a truth that should shut down the work of teaching or learning, or the work of combating ableism itself. As Katie Aubrecht writes, summarizing Roy Moodley's concept of "speaking within the sentence," we can in fact see that perhaps especially because "biomedical language and neoliberal practices [as well as "disciplinary traditions"] constrict the possibilities" for students and teachers to create change, then academia is an ideal location to interrogate these forces, an ideal place to work against ableism (Moodley, 305; Aubrecht, 190).

Ableist apologia is also related to what Shelley Tremain calls ableist exceptionism: "the phenomenon whereby values, beliefs, principles, and so on that one holds in other domains of political consciousness are not transferred over to the domain of disability and ableism" (n.p.).

For example, the "use of ableist language about disability" is assumed to be "politically neutral and innocent," defendable as just words, "despite the fact that [the speaker will] politicize virtually all other speech, identifying it as value laden and interested" (n.p.). Thus, very progressive teachers, researchers, and even activists will use words like moron or idiot even when critiquing racist, sexist, or otherwise offensive behavior, all the while refusing to admit or realize that they are channeling one form of bigotry to attack another. Their apologies tend to be particularly ironclad, as well, as their defensiveness about ableism can be protected simply by holding up the seemingly "higher" value of critiquing sexism or racism, even sometimes accusing anyone who critiques them of being racist or sexist themselves. In the end, even addressing this ableism is often impossible: it is exhausting, disheartening, deadening because one doesn't at all want to diminish the goal of fighting racism or sexism; one doesn't at all want to be accused of diminishing this fight. And yet the impact of this (defended) ableism ranges from wearying to extremely hurtful, compounded by the politics of calling it out. Sara Ahmed writes about the impact of being a "feminist killjoy": "to be willing to go against a social order, which is protected as a moral order, a happiness order is to be willing to cause unhappiness, even if unhappiness is not your cause. To be willing to cause unhappiness . . . to kill other people's joy by pointing out moments of sexism" ("Feminist," n.p.). There are similar affective dimensions, or emotional costs, to being willing to interject observations of ableism within progressive discourse, within any discourse, at any table, in any conversation. There are also powerful consequences to defending one's ableism as though it is the last thing for the progressive to care about.

This exceptionism works in the other direction as well. Because when we suggest that disability is a sort of final frontier of identity politics, we risk making the very wrong and very dangerous assumption that racism or sexism or homophobia (for example) are well understood. For instance, following the election of Donald Trump in 2016, commentators suggested that he was going to need to address the ableist comments he made about a reporter, as many Republican supporters of Trump found these comments offensive, and these people would need to be assuaged. In a famous speech at the Golden Globe Awards in early 2017, Meryl Streep repeated a variation of this story, suggesting that Trump's mocking of reporter Serge Kovaleski was particularly revealing of his poor character. But none of these commentators made any real mention of Trump's incredibly racist and sexist comments throughout his campaign, failing to argue that he would need to address and apologize for those sentiments, or that they reveal his character.

Of course, for commentators like Van Jones, the "whitelash" of the vote was in the forefront of their mind, and the election was all about race. But perhaps because disability discrimination is, in some conversations, somehow depoliticized it can be held up as a line not to cross, even while other lines are being destroyed. That is, the charitable, pitying, infantilizing view of disability somehow sensitizes people to forms of disablism or disability discrimination, while race and gender are issues of "political correctness" that are to be left untouched. But making disabled people pitiable is not somehow politically neutral; using disability as an ethical test does nothing to help us understand the connections between ableism and other forms of oppression. Ableism is never alone with itself.

So ableist exceptionism works in many directions: it could be that ableism is the only thing we won't admit is a problem; it could be that ableism is the only problem we're willing to talk about. But both reactions are of utmost importance to this book and the reactions you—as the reader—may have to it. As well as the uses you—as the reader—might make of it.

Whether any of this "talking about ableism" leads to action is another issue entirely. Because people say that "of course the university is ableist"—and this form of apologia is particularly nuanced in that it releases the person who says it from doing anything at all about this ableism. There is a shift to admitting that at the very least the university is an elitist space, but it comes joined with dismissing responsibility for doing anything about this elitism, or even interrogating its fairness. So what makes it so hard for people to both admit that the university is ableist, and to admit that this is a bad thing? What would encourage people to read a book like this without simply saying "of course there is ableism in academia" and dismissing this entire inquiry? There are certainly academics and other stakeholders who would say "of course the university is racist" and leave it at that, but it is understood that this is a response that reinforces the racism. Making this racism the center of a conversation means taking responsibility for it and committing to change. Of course it is hugely problematic to make a "like race" comparison here—but we can and should (cautiously) understand disability in a "with but not in place of race" discourse, simply because we know that ableism on college campuses is deeply racialized, as racist attitudes and practices are also ableist. Work like the landmark *Presumed Incompetent* undertakes to understand the intersecting roles of race, gender, and class in the working lives of women faculty of color. Ableism can and should often be seen as an intersecting force as well—not more than, not in place of, but always in a layered and complicated relationship with these other forms of structural discrimination.

Universities are not, for instance, less racist than they are ableist. Instead, the two forces work together, and must be addressed together. This means never forgetting or downplaying how these forces work together. This means never excusing or downplaying the ableism or the racism of the academy.

The point is to find ways to get the stakeholders in higher education to engage with, understand, and take action to address racism, classism, sexism, transphobia, ableism, and other structural inequalities, biases, and the range of harmful practices they allow. Saying "of course the university is ableist" is a first step that necessitates further action. It should not be a disaffected claim that releases one from responsibility.

Academic ableism is a difficult thing to consider. Coming to terms with ableism in higher education means questioning, as well, our own privilege, the very system that rewards professors and administrators and placed us at the top of a set of steep stairs. So let's pay attention to how ableism occurs, and when, and to whom, and to what effect, and let's pay attention to how we might resist and refuse ableism, and what else ableism is connected to in history, in theory, in practice, and through teaching and research and service. Saying "of course the university is ableist" does not defuse academic ableism. Instead, it often subtly excuses it, subconsciously submerges its roots and branches, and ends a conversation that needs to be just a beginning. This attitude of fatigue around ableism hides it under the disguise of elitism, which is viewed as a neutral or even a positive value, an excusable problem or a byproduct of the culture of universities. A kind of polite attitude about elitism is one of the most pervasive disguises for ableism. In the chapters that follow, I will provide a variety of forms of evidence, and a variety of ways to clearly think through the ableism of the university. The goal is to work straight through the resistance one might feel about ableism, to address the politeness of elitism, and to question the ways stakeholders may subconsciously protect their own privilege on their paths up and down the steep steps of academia.

CHAPTER ONE

Steep Steps

David Orr, from a recent article entitled "Architecture
as Pedagogy":

"The curriculum embedded in any building instructs as fully
and as powerfully as any course taught in it." (212)

In this chapter, I will continue to interrogate and remap the spaces and
interfaces of the North American university, analyzing the ways that
educational institutions have "limit[ed] public access and interaction
in such a way as to avoid the chance encounter of diverse populations,
creating a series of protected interior and isolated spaces" (Hardt and
Negri, 188), as well as the ways that we might more actively, inclusively
design our teaching in response to, and with an awareness of, this architecture. I will put forward three images through my first three chapters:
steep steps, the retrofit, and universal design. These three images represent spatial metaphors that come from within the field of disability
studies and nicely articulate the ways space excludes, the ways space can
be redesigned, and the ways space can be more inclusively conceived. My
criteria for selecting these metaphors is a simple one: I want them to be
readily recognizable. Teachers might experience these spaces every day
as they come to work—and not just when they encounter steps or ramps
in the approach to the classroom or studio, but also in its layout, in classroom texts, in responses to student work, in paper prompts or assign-

ments, in workshop and collaborative design, on class message boards or websites, in labs. The metaphors are also spaces that are produced, ideologically, in the world in which we move. First of all, the university erects steep steps to keep certain bodies and minds out. Secondly, to retrofit our structures for access, we add ramps at the sides of buildings and accommodations to the standard curriculum—still, disability can never come in the front entrance. But finally, in theory and practice, we can recognize the ways that teaching can be universally designed—how we might create an enabling space for learning and a way to think broadly and inclusively about ability.

With my words, I want to try and create a new map of higher education, a map that recognizes the ways students with disabilities have been excluded, the ways the academy has accommodated them, as well as the ways that disability, as an identity and an epistemology, as a way of being in the world and making meaning in the world, will continue to push us to understand teaching and learning in new, broader, and more empowering ways.

Architectures of Ableism

So the first premise of this chapter is that we need to care about space. To begin with, we do think spatially—we readily perceive the world in terms of physical space and spatial relations. Thus, spaces already convey information, and reconstructing or reimagining these spaces is an act of persuasion.

There is a phrase that many disability studies teachers have heard from colleagues over and over again, noted first by Amy Vidali who noticed how often other teachers said to her "but there are no disabled students in my class." This statement is a kind of apologia for not creating an inclusive classroom. The statement is something that Vidali and other disability scholars find sad and ironic and maybe a bit humorous: it is statistically and practically nearly impossible. The sad or scary part is that this statement sounds or feels like a wish or a desire. That wish or desire for higher education without disability is academic ableism in a nutshell, and it is rooted in eugenics, as I showed in my "approach." But by more literally mapping disability as a reality and an important, contributing population in colleges and universities, there is a move to refuse this desire for academia and for an educational space without disability.

As David Harvey and others have argued, "representations of places have material consequences insofar as fantasies, desires, fears and longings are expressed in actual behavior" *(From Space to Place* , 22). Spaces, and how we write about them, think about them and move through them, suggest and delimit attitudes. As Stewart Brand wrote in *How Buildings Learn,* the term architecture means "unchanging deep structure" (2). But this is an illusion: building "means both the action and the verb build and 'that which is built'" (2). Buildings are "always building and rebuilding. The idea is crystalline, the fact fluid" (2). Yet Rob Imrie has written about the "design apartheid" against people with disabilities— the methodical exclusion of disabled people from planning, architecture, and design decision making. This exclusion maps a wish: "there are no people with disabilities here." In this way, disabled people have been traditionally excluded both from buildings and from the ongoing building of academia. As Brendan Gleeson shows, "Disabled people in Western societies have been oppressed by the production of space . . . due in part to their exclusion from the discourses and practices that shape the physical layout of societies" (2).

Further, as Tanya Titchkosky argues, "the mapping of disability is an imparting of some version of what disability is and, thus, contains implicit directions for how to move around, through or with it. . . . disability has a long history of being mapped as if it is a foreign land, and a distanced curiosity remains one of the most repetitive, debilitating, yet 'normal' ways of regarding the life and work of disabled people" ("Cultural Maps," 101, 109). In the modern university, students with disabilities are kept far away from the discussions within which their input could be most illuminating, most challenging. This exclusion extends from dialogue to infrastructure: as Sharon Snyder and David Mitchell write, "the built environment also includes the mythologies, images and characterizations about disability that comprise the majority of interactions in our imaginary lives" (Narrative, xiv). Yet, as Snyder and Mitchell write, "we cannot know a culture until we ask its disabled citizens to assess it" (Narrative, 178). Likewise, we cannot understand academia until we interrogate it from the viewpoint of disability. Allow me to repeat myself: if rhetoric is the circulation of discourse through the body, then spaces and institutions cannot be disconnected from the bodies within them, the bodies they selectively exclude, and the bodies that actively intervene to reshape them.

As I will show, disability is a reality—in the lives of those who claim this identity and in the lives of those who believe themselves immune. Disability is also produced, sometimes most powerfully, by our uses of space. If the teacher wants to, above all, treat students ethically and respectfully, she must consider the spaces where she teaches in terms of disciplinary attitudes, but also in terms of bricks and mortar, walls and steps, and pixels and bits that exclude bodies. The disciplinary and the institutional, the discursive and the physical, must be considered always in interaction. We need to start with exclusion. While in civic planning we have premises like Henri Lefebvre's claim of a "right to the city," where the mandate of the city as a social construction is to serve all its citizens (and not only an exclusive set), academic ableism leads us to believe that in fact there are some specific bodies and minds that do not at all have a right to the university. The connected feeling is that the spaces and architectures of the university have been and should continue to be designed to filter out certain bodies and minds. The spatial metaphor for this process is the steep steps.

Again, in this chapter, there will be discussion of eugenics, rape, sexual harassment, and sexual coercion. These matters may be especially triggering for some readers as I will be discussing the ways that colleges and universities refuse responsibility, deny justice, and silence victims.

Steep Steps to Ivory Towers

The steep steps metaphor describes how the university has been constructed as a place for the very able. The steep steps metaphor puts forward the idea that access to the university is a movement upwards—only the truly "fit" survive this climb. University campuses have lots of steep steps—but the entire university experience can also be metaphorized as a movement up steep steps. The steep steps, physically and figuratively, lead to the ivory tower. The tower is built upon ideals and standards—historically, this is an identity that the university has embraced. I want to suggest that we have mapped the university in this way—as a climb up the stairs of the ivory tower—for particular reasons. Often, maps are created not to reveal exclusion, but to create it. Mapping is traditionally a mode of closing-off, of containment. Simply, maps cut people out much more than they fit people in. David Sibley, the cultural geographer who has perhaps most extensively theorized the exclusionary potential of spatialization, extends this idea of "structuring subjectivity." He writes that "space and society are implicated in the construction of the boundaries of the self but . . . the self is also projected onto society and onto space"

(86). Simply, how we want to understand ourselves affects how we construct and experience space. The way we think of ourselves is projected onto our classroom space. When someone says "there are no disabled students in my class," this is a map of fear, perhaps (access Vidali). But it is also voicing a desire. There is a fear of the presence of disability and a desire for its opposite: its eradication and exclusion. The steep steps metaphor sums up the ways the university constructs spaces that exclude. The self or selves that have been projected upon the space of the university are not just able-bodied and normal, but exceptional, elite. This projection unites many other discourses of normativity: whiteness, heteronormativity, empire, colonialism, masculinity. In connected ways, these discourses push down and mark some bodies while insisting on the natural, unmarked place of the privileged at the top of the steps. The same thing happens, often concurrently, with the marking of minds. The university pulls some people slowly up the stairs, and it arranges others at the bottom of this steep incline. The university also steps our society, reinforcing hierarchies and divisions. For instance, as previously mentioned, people with disabilities have been traditionally seen as objects of study in higher education, rather than as teachers or students. Disability has been a rhetorically produced stigma that could be applied to other marginalized groups to keep them out of the university (and away from access to resources and privileges).

The steps work as well to teach students to look down upon those on the steps below them while they carefully maintain their own positions. As Carol Schick argues in an essay entitled "Keeping the Ivory Tower White," white students' "bourgeois white identification relies on their allegiance to prestigious white space and their access to privilege and social respectability. They depend on university processes," even those designed to create a tokenized "diversity" to "support white domination so that they may establish and produce their own legitimacy as 'good' teaching bodies and 'respectable' Canadian citizens" (Schick, 119). To put this in more simple terms, white students know that the fakeness and ineffectiveness of diversity initiatives on campus maintain their white privilege sometimes just as powerfully as overt forms of discrimination do. If white students play along with the pantomime of tokenized diversity, they won't have to challenge their own privilege or lose their own positioning.

Similarly, allegiance to a respectable form of ableist rhetoric—or ableist apologia—is required of faculty and students if they hope to access the privilege of the university themselves. If faculty and students can be seen to just try to accommodate some of the time, to play along with the game of accessibility and inclusion, they know that their own intelligence, ways of learning, and embodiment can be kept safe from stigmatization, can be unaltered and unexamined. Students and teachers will show allegiance to exclusions that reinforce their privilege, and show allegiance to processes that maintain it. It is not just in assessment situations in the classroom in which teachers are asked to decide who gets to be included and who does not—this selection is folded into every aspect of university life. Ableism is not a series of bad or sad anomalies, a series of discrete actions. It is a rhetoric in the fullest sense of the word: gestural, social, architectural, duplicitous and plain, malleable, and immovable. And it requires agents. It requires actions and intentional inaction.

It seems as though, regardless of the architectural style(s) of a campus, steep steps are integral, whether these are the wide marble staircases of Greek-revival administration buildings and "approaches," or the brutalist concrete stairs and terraces like those constructed on my own campus at the University of Waterloo. The most traditional of campuses, many of them built around churches, or in classical Ionic style, similarly rely on steps not just as architectural details but as symbolic social centerpieces of university life—traditional university life. For example, think of Amory Blaine in F. Scott Fitzgerald's *This Side of Paradise*. He develops a "deep and reverent devotion to the gray walls and Gothic peaks [of Princeton] and all they symbolized as warehouses of dead ages. . . . he liked knowing that Gothic architecture, with its upward trend, was peculiarly appropriate" to his elite university (62). This same upward trend builds stairs, as well as some peculiar attitudes about who can come within the walls, and who can ascend the heights, and who deserves to be on the upper steps. Unsurprisingly, when Disney/Pixar animators wanted to create a realistically forbidding setting for the film *Monsters University*, they studied several Ivy League schools: the MU School of Scaring has broad, high marble stairs just like those you'd find at Harvard or Stanford.[1] In reality, and in the public imagination, higher education is about steep steps. I will also return to the metaphorical message sent by the Monsters U. gates, themselves modeled after those on exclusive campuses like Berkeley and Harvard.

They are onto something. Using gates as ideological foci—or the main visual focus—of college architecture has traditionally ensured that we will view the university as set apart from society. Ironically, the same gates were built and used in other "total institutions" like asylums to forcibly keep the public out and the deviant in; college gates keep the public out and the elite in. Further, the gates urge us to understand academia as a space to protect and as a space to be "secured." This securing means that an African-American professor such as Ursula Ore, as Jennifer Doyle points out, can be subject to carding—a demand to "show her papers" or identification—on campus. When Ore refused this request, she was physically restrained, cuffed, straddled against a police car, and later charged with assault. This fear of interlopers is also what led to the repeated tasering of Mostafa Tobatabainejad in a UCLA library in 2006. He was a student, in his library, studying—but was rendered suspect because of his ethnicity, and the situation escalated. In Canada, as Sandy Hudson points out, "It would be very difficult for you to find a university or college aged black person who hasn't had some kind of experience with carding" on campus (Miranda, n.p.).[2] As Doyle reminds us, carding or "ID checks are all too common for black and brown students, faculty, and staff" (Doyle, 58). This securing also leads, as Morgan Holmes has shown, to "discipline" in the form of campus bans for students with mental illness or psychological disabilities. In Holmes's words, there is "a trajectory toward removal of students who do not 'fit in' because they have a medical diagnosis" (n.p.). At the same time, schools fail to "protect students from their [sexual] assailants on campus. In other words, in a world where sexual assault is normal but "Asperger" is not, a rapist is not subject [to this trajectory towards removal] but a student with ASD is" (Holmes, n.p.). A student who has been a victim of rape can assume that their rapist will remain on campus and may need to do something as extraordinary as carrying a mattress around campus for a year in order to call attention to this—as Emma Sulkowicz did at Columbia University (access Mitra's review of Sulkowicz). Yet a student of color can assume that an ordinary part of campus life will include university security questioning their right to be there in ways that call attention to their difference.

So, the ongoing policing of the inside and the outside of higher education ensures a state of campus (in)security that almost always plays itself out on a certain set of bodies. For instance, as Leila Whitley and Tiffany Page show in an article in the journal *New Formations*,

> after 31 current and former University of California Berkeley students filed two federal complaints against the university alleging the mishandling of sexual assault investigations, a review of four California universities conducted by the California State Auditor found that in more than half of the cases reviewed the universities could not demonstrate that complainants were informed of investigation out-

comes. . . . institutional quiet becomes yet another means, among the institutional and legal frameworks . . . to enable sexism to remain out of sight, to conceal behaviour and to return the institution to a normalised state of affairs." (n.p.)

In other words, as a newspaper article in the *Guardian* stated in its title: "In Academia, There Is No Such Thing as Winning a Sexual Harassment Complaint" (Postgraduate).

In a very separate and yet somehow similar scenario in this same California system, a campus police officer was caught pepper-spraying nonviolent student protestors at UC Davis. It wasn't enough that the police were dressed in riot gear, armed, and felt that pepper-spraying was the most effective way to deal with a student protest, but the university subsequently spent $175,000 to "scrub" mentions of this incident from the Internet, to ensure that no one searching "UC Davis" would access this news.

With the university most interested in protecting itself and its reputation, in Jennifer Doyle's words, "We swap out teaching for securitization—for the internalization within every student of [the] sense of being always-already-in-violation that defines the entire campus" and that particularly defines and is defined by legalistic logics such as accommodation (Doyle, 116). The campus is "a private zone that must be protected from the "non-affiliate," from public invasion" (Doyle 44). The campus ostensibly gets walled-off to protect students. This also protects and prolongs and provides grounds for practices of surveillance and segmentation that would never be allowed in the "real world." Further, the university hides ableism behind idealism. As Holmes argues, "We are damaging one kind of health in the name of a perniciously normative health, then, at all stages of what was meant to be a public good" (n.p.). Staying silent about harassment and rape, squashing negative press, these things are done to protect education and educators, who we assume to be good. But these moves put students in danger, constructing every student as a possible threat to the reputation of the school. This extends to the legalization of the accommodation process for disabled students—the student is seen as someone who must be prevented from suing the school, and this is in part already a liability. The gates, towers, and steep steps should make us understand how deeply these architectural investments imprint educational attitudes: who gets kept out, who and what gets held carefully within, and what conduct can be excused, which rights can be suspended, on campus?

Eugenic Mergers

As mentioned in my "approach," another way to map the spaces of academia and disability would be to look at the ways land was parceled out in the United States in the early to mid-1800s. While land-grant universities were popping up in rural spaces, asylums were popping up in other, nearby rural settings—on old farms and abandoned land. Yet the two institutions were often tightly hinged or merged together. From within one privileged space, academics were deciding the fate of others in similar, yet somehow now pathological, other, and impure spaces. Or, as Zosha Stuckey has shown, you have huge institutions like the New York State Asylum for Idiots, "rhetorically" educating young people just down the road from Syracuse University. My own alma mater, Miami University of Ohio, is a school that traces its origins to 1809, and at first glance seems to have a strong tradition of creating academic subjects, not academic objects. Yet, as is the case with many, many North American universities, Miami shared land with an institution of connected, but inverse intentions—a sanitarium for the treatment of mental disorders. To understand the contemporary state of "campus security," mentioned above, we have to connect to this longer history.

As Henry Howe wrote in 1888, "Oxford [Ohio, home of Miami University] is purely a college town: and its various institutions are each in localities with pleasant outlooks. Among them is a sanitarium, the 'Oxford Retreat,' a private institution for the treatment of nervous diseases and insanity. Through its ample grounds winds a little stream" (355). Beside the building were formal gardens, and in these gardens, in 1905, "the first [Miami University] Junior Prom was held . . . the couples strolling past a flock of stately peacocks on the autumn grounds" (Havighurst, 165). The flip side of this charming outward appearance was that the Retreat was a place of secure isolation; streams and peacocks and formally dressed undergrads promenading on the outside, patients locked inside. Dr. Cook, the owner of the Retreat, built an underground tunnel from his home to the building, to enable him to travel from building to building "without being seen by his patients" (Havighurst, 158). At the Retreat, Dr. Cook also performed lobotomies and shock treatments.

You may have also seen a recent news item about the University of Mississippi discovering a graveyard on land it was clearing to build a Medical Center. In clearing the land, they found over 1,000 unmarked graves, believed to be those of patients at the former Mississippi State Lunatic Asylum (access Jerry Mitchell). The shock registered in news stories seemed to be associated with the fact that this discovery would halt the construction, and there is definitely a little bit of drama invoked in articles about the discovery, mentioning the idea of "ghosts" and "haunting" and a "horror movie." But nowhere is there any real outrage or horror about the fact that these graves were unmarked, that these patients weren't deemed deserving of a proper burial, that these lives were so demeaned. You could look to nearly any major state university and find similar links. For instance, there is another controversy about unmarked graves (and nearly 100 bodies unaccounted for) at the former State Colony for the Feebleminded in Austin, Texas, just a mile away from the University of Texas. Again, the controversy seems to be more about the value of land (estimated to be worth $25 million) adjacent to the university, and not about those who died.

These connections reveal, first of all, the steady pattern of setting up such sites of incarceration in close proximity to universities, where one group of humans could be held and studied by another. One can also recognize what the binary relationship has always been between universities and hospitals and asylums like these. What a statement to the future doctors who will be trained at this medical center in Mississippi, for instance. Their learning now literally unfolds upon an ignorance of the eugenic past. Perhaps the most perverse instantiation of the logic of the steep steps we might hope to find is revealed: we continue to actually build universities in service of and on top of the history of eugenics, lifting some bodies upwards toward privilege upon the footings of segregation and oppression.

Places like the Oxford Retreat were labs for the development of negative eugenics—the destruction of supposedly inferior "stock" through isolation and sterilization. Many children from large immigrant families were shipped to these institutions, in both Canada and the United States, and there was a radically disproportionate number of African Americans, Eastern Europeans, and lower-class children, all expendable according to eugenic thinking. Miami University and other colleges, on the other hand, might be seen as an arena for positive eugenics, the propagation of (supposedly) superior "stock." As Charles Murray has shown, North American colleges and universities have been tremendously successful at sorting citizens, with the top 10 U.S. schools sucking up 20 percentage of the top group of students—based on standardized tests. This sorting then also leads to what he calls "cognitive homogamy: when individuals with similar cognitive ability have children" (61). What could be more eugenic than this? Yet we act like this is some sort of accident. It is not.

To this day Miami maintains the robust "Miami Merger" program, sending Valentine's Day cards and promotional materials to every individual who met their spouse at Miami, boasting that "out of 151,967 living alums, 24,882 are married to each other, creating 12,441 "Miami Mergers." That's about 16.4 percent of Miami's alumni population" ("News Briefs").

My partner and I married while we were both graduate students at Miami. Thus, we weren't actually Miami mergers, but for one year we were treated as such. In 2005, we were mailed a magnet distributed to couples on Valentine's Day to promote the merger program. The magnet had a slightly blurry image of a white male and female couple kissing in an archway on campus. Over the image there was a poem printed: "Here's a magnet you take apart, to become a picture frame and a heart. Display it with a photo inside. You're a Miami Merger, show it with pride!" The words Miami and Merger were printed in larger, red letters, above and below this image and poem. Beside this was the above-mentioned photo frame, which could be clicked out of the magnet so that you could place your own "merger" photo inside. The magnet also said "Happy Valentine's Day 2005" and, at the bottom, "from the Miami Alumni Association."

There should be a visceral sense of disconnection between the poetry on the card and the eugenic segregation (and research) we have witnessed throughout history. The Miami Retreat and the Miami Merger represent two extremes: one group of people institutionalized out of the gene pool, one group coerced into the gene pool. Negative eugenics could not be more clearly set in contrast to positive eugenics. It is also impossible to disconnect the idea of the merger from the reality of rape culture on campuses—especially a campus where, in 2012, a flier was found listing the "top ten ways to get away with rape" (Jones).

A quick aside: I will discuss this rape culture on college campuses in greater depth later in the book, but for the purposes of this first chapter, all about steep steps and ivory towers, we should note the title of Bonnie Fisher, Leah Daigle, and Francis Cullen's landmark book on the topic of campus rape: *Unsafe in the Ivory Tower: The Sexual Victimization of College Women*. In the book, they show that one-fifth to one-quarter of women at U.S schools will be victims of rape or attempted rape. In Canada, because of a lack of similar research, universities are expected to self-report. Upsettingly, but perhaps unsurprisingly, this allows schools to drastically underreport or even hide the truth. Canadian schools would have us believe that "for 2014, the total number of alleged incidents of sexual assault reported to campus authorities amounted to 1.85 per 10,000 students." As the CBC (Canada's national broadcaster) argues, this "is well below what many researchers believe is the case" (Ward). There is likewise little research into sexual assault against students with disabilities, though we know that 83 percent of disabled women will be sexually assaulted in their lifetime, a shocking statistic. The only current study on campus prevalence, by Gwendolyn Francavillo into the experience of Deaf and hard-of-hearing students, suggested that 48% of these students experienced unwanted sexual contact, at least double the rate of hearing students in the United States. In short, rape and sexual assault are themselves a force for disablement on college campuses. Students with disabilities are disproportionately impacted.

As an "alum" of Miami of Ohio, a school where, in my first year on campus, a cross was burned on a town lawn and a hateful e-mail was sent to LGBTQ2 students who listed their names in the campus paper on national coming-out day, I feel uncomfortable about the message sent by the picture of a white heterosexual couple embracing on the "merger" magnet (Nasty E-mail). The intention is not to attack Miami, which is certainly (and scarily) no different in its legacy than many other schools. But we need to locate a common and insistent theme in North American academia. There are many other "merger" programs like this one, and couples who met on campus are specific targets of fundraisers. At Loyola University Chicago, there are "Rambler Romances"; at American University in Washington, there is a "Sweethearts" program. As fundraising consultants point out, "If you have both partners in a relationship that graduated from the same university, you have a better chance of getting gifts and getting bigger gifts over time" ("Miami Mergers," n.p.). These mergers, then, often take on an economic connotation: the best eugenic stock meets one another on campus, combines their worth, and then contributes back to the school, thus further shaping it in their image and with their dollars. As Elizabeth Duffy's 1998 *Crafting a Class* showed, admissions policies are often focused on the potential of students to later become donors. It is a positive eugenic dream come true, especially in an era of real college mergers—when the have-not schools are literally forced to combine with one another to stay alive because of the public defunding of education, and the most affluent institutions continue to attract a tremendous amount of donated money, privately. More and more, they invest this money dubiously.[3] What these economics show is that the steep steps have strong historical roots: they were created in part by the parceling out of land and the juxtaposition of spaces of higher learning beside spaces of warehousing and experimentation. The steep steps also continue to grow steeper: privilege begets privilege. Finally: eugenics is alive, well, and hard at work at North American colleges and universities.

Building Disability

The argument I am making here is that, basically, academia exhibits and perpetuates a form of structural ableism. I borrow to a certain degree from the notion of structural racism, defined by the Aspen Institute as follows:

> A system in which public policies, institutional practices, cultural representations, and other norms work in various, often reinforcing ways to perpetuate racial group inequity. It identifies dimensions of our history and culture that have allowed privileges associated with "whiteness" and disadvantages associated with "color" to endure and adapt over time. Structural racism is not something that a few people or institutions choose to practice. Instead it has been a feature of the social, economic and political systems in which we all exist. (n.p.)

Likewise, ableism has to be seen as a series of entrenched structures—not just the action of an individual or of individuals. We have to understand that because of these pervasive structures, we live in a society that resists efforts to ameliorate or get rid of ableism. As scholar and activist Daniel Freeman writes, "Able-bodied people all have things that they fall short with, skills or tasks that they will never master. But when disabled folks say, 'These are the things I need in order to do my very best,' it is labeled as an 'accommodation.' . . . The language itself is ableist in nature, bringing into focus the reality of how disabled bodies are seen as barriers to able-bodied life" (n.p.). Accommodation is thought of as something that always needs to be created, something that has a cost. This underlines the inherent inaccessibility of nearly all of society: seemingly, nothing is ever designed to be accessible in the first place. Accessibility itself is an exnomination, a negative or inverse term, existentially second to inaccessibility. Accessibility is existentially second in a way that demands a body that cannot access. Nothing is inaccessible until the first body can't access it, demands access to it, or is recognized as not having access. As the great philosopher of disability Tobin Siebers wrote, "when a disabled body moves into any space, it discloses the social body implied by that space. There is a one-to-one correspondence between the dimensions of the built environment and its preferred social body—the body invited inside as opposed to those bodies not issued an invitation" (85). In this way, the structural ableism of society mandates not just that structures be built only for preferred bodies, but that this preferred status be borne out and proven by all of the bodies that are denied access. Having access, then, is not momentous for those who can easily move through these spaces. Being denied access—and pointing out this denial—creates a spectacle. Needing access is momentous.

But what does it mean, then, to suggest that disability is constructed? As I have written before, an emphasis on social construction can often defuse the political power of an identity group. Social constructionism, in some ways, can be used as a method of silencing. Particularly, social construction can remove the focus on the particularity of differences of bodies and minds—if we are all disabled by an oppressive environment or architecture or pedagogy in some way, why does the disability perspective really matter? How is the embodied experience of disability any different from the norm? The final effect can often be just as oppressive as the reality that social construction serves to critique. Without the solidarity and political unity that come with disability identity, it is very difficult to challenge the norm. But a cautious and rights-oriented social constructionist philosophy can interrogate or explore the ways that bodies and cultures, biology and social structures—even texts—interact and cocreate one another.

To explore this cautious interrogation, let's look at one particular example: the ways that buildings, in the last three decades, have increasingly been understood as capable of making people sick.

Sick buildings were made possible by certain economic conditions: architects could create airtight and efficient buildings with open floor plans because of "conditions of relative privilege and luxury" (Murphy, 3). There was "an expectation of comfort and safety as conditions of daily life" and yet also "a sense that privilege was imperfect, even threatened": the very conditions of privilege could be toxic (Murphy, 3). These airtight buildings also circulated toxins. The creation of "sick buildings" is an example of the ways that architecture can actually disable. As Michelle Murphy writes, "the making of office buildings, homes, and other seemingly innocuous places into sites where chemical exposures occurred or did not occur was among other things an effect of power, power than could only be exercised on uneven terrain" (178).

Murphy continues:

> When the toxic effect of the vast majority of chemicals remained untested, when exposures themselves regularly escaped detection, people who believed their bodies were reacting to the background noise of everyday chemicals had very little secure knowledge from which to begin coping with their afflictions. . . . the struggle by ordinary people to understand their bodies and the consequential, sometimes deliberate, undermining of their effort resonates with a political, and not just poignant, valence. (178)

The phenomena of sick buildings became a drama of perceptibility and imperceptibility, a constant debate about "is it real or not?" (18). The drama or debate connects both directly and metaphorically to academic ableism. First of all, many universities contain sick buildings: a simple Google search turns up hundreds of examples of the spread of viruses because of poor ventilation, mold, and so on; as well as cases of exposure to dangerous chemicals both directly and acutely, and slowly, over time on campuses. But the power dynamics around the ways that college campuses make students sick are also similar in many ways to the power dynamics around how college campuses disable. For instance, while we think we know (and we argue, over and over again, that we know) what the benefits of an education are, what are its harms? Who can expose these harms? Why is this exposure so difficult? As Murphy argues, "The imperceptibility and uncertainty of such harms can be the tangible, and even purposeful, result of human action" in the case of sick buildings (180). That is, it is not just the sickness of the buildings that is a human product, it is also the very difficulty of exposing this sickness that is the result of intentional action.

We can say that illness and disability are constructed by these buildings, very literally. Yet who claims this construction matters, as does the fact that college processes are designed—yes, constructed—to deny claims of sickness and disability or to deny responsibility for them. What does it mean to suggest that disability is in part socially constructed? In one sense, it means that those who expose these realities might be blamed for them or disbelieved as the university secures itself.

There are other ways that universities create sickness, of course. A 2015 study at the University of California at Berkeley found that 47 percent of graduate students suffer from depression, following from a 2005 study that showed 10 percent had contemplated suicide (Fogg). A 2003

Australian study found that the rate of mental illness in academic staff was three to four times higher than in the general population (Winefield et al.). According to a *New Scientist* article, the percentage of academics with mental illness in the United Kingdom has been estimated at 53 percent (Wilcox). A study by Gail Kinman and Siobhan Wray also showed that "compared to other professionals and community samples, academic staff experience less job satisfaction and extremely low levels of psychological health" (492). In no other profession is this stress better camouflaged behind other, supposedly inviolable, and more important "values" like autonomy, flexibility, and creativity. The result is a sort of boutique stress: faculty and staff may willingly or unwittingly trade in their happiness and "balance."

The social construction of disability on campus often mandates that disability exist only as a negative, private, individual failure. Very little real space is made for the building of coalitional, collective, or interdependent disability politics. Moreover, the university can never be viewed as the space responsible for causing disability. Disability had to exist prior to, has to remain external to, and has to be remedied according to the arm's-length accommodations of a blameless and secure academic institution.

Sickness and Wellness

The "sickness" model of higher education also comes into conflict with the "wellness" model. As mentioned previously, we can draw a (sort of straight) line from eugenic mental hygiene and physical fitness tests, to their existence as promotional programs, to family life education programs, to wellness initiatives. Such programs currently offload the responsibility for "wellness" onto individual students (and teachers). Eat better. Exercise more. Sleep well. (Maybe even wear this complimentary watch to track all this.) The programs often synch with "mental health awareness" on campuses—those programs that often refuse to address mental illness as a systemic issue, as something caused by college, and definitely refuse to address mental disability. What these programs also do not attempt to do is attempt to address structural ableism and the educational construction of disability. They also tend to be placed where psychologists can gather large amounts of data from a captive population—which is why so many wellness programs are helmed by psychologists or run out of psychology departments. The euphemism "wellness" also works rhetorically to demand that we do not discuss disability, especially mental illness/mental disability/madness. We now have a growing industry of professionals working to minimize and hide disability on campuses.[4] But the idea of wellness has also had an invasive effect, working its way into all aspects of university life. The most recent evidence of this trend was a "wellness agreement" that a Canadian student had to sign. A Mount Saint Vincent University student was forced to sign an agreement "forbidding him to tell other students in residence that he was feeling suicidal" (Silva). The exact language from the agreement was that the student "will not discuss or engage in conversations with residence students regarding personal issues, namely the student's self-destructive thoughts" (Silva). The penalty for breaking this contract would have been expulsion from residence.

Wellness programs, then, might be defined as contemporary "opportunity structures" for forms of eugenic thinking. An "opportunity structure" names the conditions or factors that might empower people to create social movements (and enable other changes). A university-wide program, harnessing the communications and PR power of the school, can be a particularly powerful, authoritative, legitimizing opportunity structure. In this case, the focus on wellness might provide the rhetorical conditions in which eugenic ideas about who is and is not "fit" for college can germinate and grow.

As Catherine Gidney's book *Tending the Student Body* shows, "by the 1930s and '40s, many universities provided some type of health service, and required physical examination and physical training. . . . educators had come to perceive bodily health to be a crucial component in the role of the university in shaping students' character. . . . In other words, character would become writ on the body" (15, 76). Gidney goes on to show that "anxieties about women's ability to combine intense study with good health in general, and reproductive health in particular [was] prominent within Canadian universities" (16). And, "in the late nineteenth century, some American universities, particularly elite ones, instituted compulsory medical examinations as part of their admission process in order to eliminate the unfit" (23). Unsurprisingly, "in obtaining funding for health services, physicians and administrators also relied on the help of faculty whose research intersected with aspects of the student physical examinations. . . . Physicians and scientists, and even the occasional entrepreneur, quickly identified such programs as potential sources of captive research subjects. The provision of health services in the interests of students thus blurred with the use of students as research subjects" (32).

These programs are no longer explicitly mandatory, unless you are forced to sign an agreement. Yet physicians and scientists on your campus likely study student wellness and publish about wellness without ever asking for student consent. Further, all students at Oral Roberts University are required to wear Fitbit watches to track their weight, sleep, and exercise and many university employees can earn insurance discounts by submitting to wellness checks, using wellness apps, or wearing smart watches to track themselves. And "wellness" is a theme that pervades the university through awareness days, exercise-a-thons, special yoga classes, the use of university-wide health statistics by researchers, and so on. In the sickness model, we are unsure of exactly to what degree the university might be disabling, but the blame and the impact almost always falls on individuals to shoulder. In the wellness model, we are sure we should all be physically improving on campus, not talking about disability, and the burden is on the individual student to never be unwell.

So we have the impossible challenge of *Academic Ableism*: not just to recognize where and how ableism happens, but to ask what the impact will be of exposing it, what the cost might be of assigning blame, and what the forces are that make it imperceptible, what the euphemisms are that disguise it, and how it comes to be normalized, even valorized in academia.

What if higher education isn't creating knowledge and ability but instead is systematically disabling? Or, perhaps less stridently or controversially: What if higher education constructs both knowledge and disability? What if these constructions rely on one another? Finally, if disability is in part socially constructed by academia, how do we feature and highlight the constructions that make space for agency, community, solidarity, and resilience?

Climbing the Steep Steps

Of course, disabled people have been fighting against academic ableism for decades. The very first Disabled Students Program, run by students with disabilities to provide self-advocacy, began at the University of California at Berkeley in 1970. Reacting to the history of the forced institutionalization of people with disabilities, the first Center for Independent Living was also created at Berkeley in 1972. The Individuals with Disabilities Education Act was then passed in 1975, Disability Rights Education and Defense Fund offices were started in Berkeley and Washington,

DC, in 1979, and the Americans with Disabilities Act was finally passed in 1990. Throughout this time, boycotts, sit-ins, and civil disobedience became ways to draw attention to the educational barriers facing many people with disabilities. For instance, a group of protesters staged a very physical protest against the steep steps that kept disabled people disenfranchised within legal and political processes, by taking off their braces, getting out of their wheelchairs, putting down their crutches, and climbing the Capitol Steps in Washington.

The following image, of the March 1990 ADAPT protest calling for passage of the Americans with Disabilities Act (ADA), shows the perspective of those crawling up the steps, the gravity of the metaphor, and the power of people's reaction to it.[5] Here, observing a political protest enacted over a physical (and highly symbolic) space nicely articulates my point about the alloy of architecture and ideology, the union of bodies and discourses, and it shows how powerfully the disability community has always felt about the exclusiveness of steep steps.[6]

The image depicts a view from the bottom of the steps, looking up to the Capitol Building. The steps seem very steep. We view two individuals, one crawling forward up the stairs, with his or her back to us. The other individual, a young black woman in the foreground, seems to be moving up the steps backward, one step at a time. Her torso is facing us, but her head is turned around in the other direction, looking up the steps. There is a photographer further up the steps taking a picture as well.

The disabled students' movement at schools like Berkeley in the 1970s was both part of a large ideological shift, as it was also part of a huge demographic shift—there were new immigrant groups entering college, as well as many veterans of the Vietnam War, and many veterans of the political action against this war. These people now turned some attention to the class war that American universities had been complicit in, and argued that higher education should be a civil right (access Joseph Shapiro's No Pity).

The central tenets of the disability rights movement have been pride in disability identity, collective self-representation, and a concentrated effort to remove barriers to access, perhaps most remarkably those barriers that have kept people with disabilities out of social institutions like universities. Central to this history has been the idea that disability is created by a social, physical, and educational environment shaped in ways that exclude. Eugenics works to strongly ground inferences about social worth in biological formulae, using science to suggest that differences between people are predetermined, genetic, and immutable. But

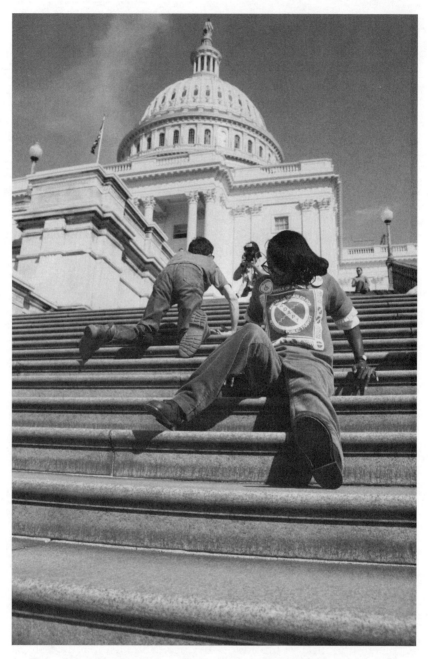

Fig. 2. Tom Olin, "Day in Court for Americans with Disabilities Protests Planned over Supreme Court's ADA Rulings." March 1990. Reprinted with permission.

what if, instead of the idea that nature determines individual success, we saw the world as inequitably shaped and built, and believed instead that the reform of society and culture would allow for a more equitable world? The social model of disability has been central to the struggle for disability rights, drawing attention to the oppression of people with disabilities. This model posits that disability is purely social, an oppression stacked onto people on top of their impairments, which are real. That said, this was largely a materialist movement, and suggests a clear bifurcation. The view was, as Michael Oliver wrote, "disablement is nothing to do with the body, impairment is nothing less than a description of the body" (34).[7] This view, applied to education, follows the hopeful model of "universal education"—believing that, given access, anyone can learn and, more broadly, suggesting that the university is the place to elevate society based on the education of all of its citizens, rather than a place to sort society based on the education of the privileged few.

In the wake of the disability rights movement, the public began to understand disability as something that is at least partially a product of the inaccessible structure of attitudes and institutions. It follows that, when we can address the cultural oppression of people with disabilities, and when we can change the way our institutions are structured and operate, we can positively affect the lives of people with disabilities (and all people, as we will all become disabled at some point in our lives).

Creating Steep Steps

Unfortunately, following the ADA, and a fairly large public backlash against this act, access for people with disabilities is no longer seen primarily as a civil rights issue.[8] Access is constructed as a matter of compliance, as the dominant terminology of the ADA is the idea of "reasonable accommodation." The "reason" of the medical and legal establishment, then, finally decides upon which accommodations are to be made—and this is reproduced at the university, where the student with disabilities must catalogue their deficits, and then is granted access through a finite range of legally and institutionally sanctioned accommodations, doled out carefully by professors and instructors under pressure and circumscription of the law. The dynamic, then, forgets the eugenic history in which those in power within the university controlled the lives of people with disabilities, positioning themselves as the arbiters of ability.[9] The dynamic also asks us to continue to favor the educational philosophy that the university is a place to sort society based on the education of the "deserving" few, rather than as the place to elevate society based on the education of all of its citizens.

Making disability seem inimical to or out of place at the university has been a strategy used to shore up the identity of those invested in higher education: if those who do not "qualify" can be vilified, marked out, and kept away, then those who make it up the stairs must deserve to. In this way, the university disavows disability—the steep steps create an environment in which disability cannot be validated or recognized, in which students with disabilities must fall to the bottom. The fall or the sorting occurs because, over time, those invested in higher education have refused to believe that the body traversing the steps could be disabled, that the elite mind could be imperfect. At the same time, their legitimate fears, perhaps grown from the realization of their own weaknesses, their own vulnerability, led to the creation of disability as a kind of counterimage. Of course, the reality is that disability is always present—there is no perfect body or mind. There is no normal body or mind. In North America, one-fifth of the population is disabled. We live in an age when, despite physical/medical efforts to avoid it and psychological/medical efforts to disavow and pathologize it, we will all become disabled at some point in our lives. I'll repeat this, asking you to remove any of the dread that might be programmed into the phrase, culturally: we will all become disabled at some point in our lives. Disavowing disability is in no body's best interest.

Teachers recognize the diversity of the students they teach. But teachers must also recognize their roles within institutions, disciplines, and perhaps even personal pedagogical agendas, in which they may seek to avoid and disavow the very idea of disability—to give it no place. This avoidance and disavowal brings with it its own spatial metaphors—I use the steep steps to express this negative force. That these steps are real in the lives of people with disabilities adds to the power of the metaphor. The steps have a strong connotation in the disability community, and not just for people who use wheelchairs and crutches. When I say that the academy builds steep steps, I hope that this verb entails many things— most of all, I want to show that the steep steps are constructed for a reason. As I have already shown, not only did eugenics actually reshape the North American population through things like immigration restriction, not only did it reshape families through its campaigns for "better breeding," not only did it reshape bodies through medical reinvention, but it reshaped how North Americans thought about bodies and minds.

Here, for example, is a diagram of the steps that were created to distinguish between different grades of the "feeble-minded" in the United States in the heyday of the eugenics movement before the Second World War. The definitions were used to classify a group of humans according to mental age, suggesting that development had been arrested and would proceed no further past the step at which the individual was placed. The mental age was determined based upon variations of a standard test, the Binet test, which asked literally hundreds of standard common-knowledge questions, of increasing difficulty. The test was also designed to stop the subject once they had reached the stage or step of difficulty at which they could proceed no further.

This image shows five people, each stationed on one of five very steep steps. The bottom person, slouched on the ground, is labeled an "idiot, mentally 3 yrs. old." On the next step up, an individual is hunched over, looking downwards, labeled "low-grade imbecile, 4 to 5 yrs. old." Next step up, a "medium imbecile, mentally 6 to 8 yrs. old." Then a "high grade imbecile, mentally 8 to 10 yrs. Old" is pictured on the next step up, now gazing upwards. Finally, we view a person, described in the caption as a "moron, mentally 10 to 12 years old," attempting to climb above the final and topmost step but only getting halfway up.

As the image reveals, the steps were also closely associated with forms of work, and thus classed citizens and linked their value to this labor-output, but also placed almost all of the feebleminded below reason and judgment, not only in a space of rational vacuity, but deficit. You'll also notice that the bodily bearing of these individuals conveys a message: the different levels of animation suggest physical and cognitive correlation. These people look tired. The disabled mind equates with the disabled body. These states correspond with affects: the slumped shoulders and downcast eyes suggest or physicalize depression.

If these steps in the image on the next page represent the very bottom of the steep set we climb to the ivory tower, they nonetheless cannot be disconnected from the history of North American higher education. In fact, "morons," "imbeciles," and "idiots" were both rhetorically (and eugenically) constructed by the "fathers" of higher education, and those individuals who were given these labels were also studied and researched.[10] At the top of the steps were those who taught and studied at premier universities, and these people studied and experimented upon the bodies of those on the bottom steps.

We may like to believe that, today, practices of eugenics have not only been rejected but that they've also been corrected. Yet the selectivity of

EXHIBIT OF WORK AND EDUCATIONAL CAMPAIGN FOR JUVENILE MENTAL DEFECTIVES

Between October 7 and 13, moving pictures at the Metropolitan Insurance Building will show the work for mentally defective children which the New York Department of Public Charities has undertaken through its clearing house for mental defectives. Started as an experiment the first of January, 1913, this clearing house has already proved its worth in meeting an actual need. Hitherto there has been no place where the mental condition of child or adult could be determined by scientifically trained experts and officially recorded for future reference and comparison.

Now, clinics in charge of Dr. Max Schlapp, seven assistant neurologists and three psychologists, held for the present at the Post Graduate Hospital, are receiving children from juvenile courts, from the Society for the Prevention of Cruelty to Children, from churches and settlements—in all, from 147 different individual sources, and are giving each child the best possible examination.

Binet tests. Reports are then sent to the organization from which the child came together with recommendations for treatment.

About 2800 such examinations have been made. The results are recorded by stenographers present at the clinic. These records are, of course, confidential and will be open for study only to accredited investigators. The facts will be confirmed by each child's finger print, to aid in any future identification and comparison of data.

Strange to say, strong opposition to institutional treatment comes often from

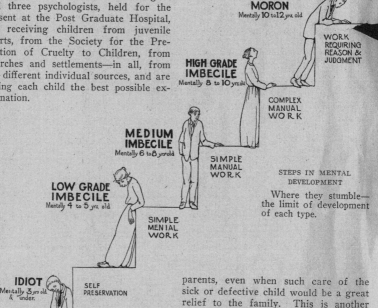

MORON
Mentally 10 to 12 yrs old

WORK
REQUIRING
REASON &
JUDGMENT

HIGH GRADE
IMBECILE
Mentally 8 to 10 yrs old

COMPLEX
MANUAL
WORK

MEDIUM
IMBECILE
Mentally 6 to 8 yrs old

SIMPLE
MANUAL
WORK

STEPS IN MENTAL
DEVELOPMENT

Where they stumble—
the limit of development
of each type.

LOW GRADE
IMBECILE
Mentally 4 to 5 yrs old

SIMPLE
MENIAL
WORK

IDIOT
Mentally 3 yrs old
& under.

SELF
PRESERVATION

The child's family history is sought, his antecedents and the influence surrounding his first years; any physical defects, such as defective teeth, adenoids, eye or ear trouble are noted and an examination made of personal tendencies and mental efficiency by the

parents, even when such care of the sick or defective child would be a great relief to the family. This is another proof of the need for a campaign of education of parents. Such education will be advanced in part by the nurses who visit the homes in an attempt to ensure the treatment recommended. It is hoped that the suitability and resources of Randall's Island as a place of retreat for children needing skilled care, may be increased and developed by adequate appropriation of funds.

Fig. 3. "Exhibit of Work and Educational Campaign for Juvenile Mental Defectives." American Philosophical Society, 1906.

this environment must be continually interrogated or questioned. We must all evaluate the ways in which we ourselves continue to decide which bodies and which minds will have access to the considerable resources, privileges, and advantages we have and we bestow—and as we ask this question, we must wonder whether what we have to offer is truly worthwhile if it translates into policies of exclusion, programs of incarceration, and reductive definitions of human worth.

Interrogating the steep steps metaphor works to highlight not just how space and spatialization are exclusionary but also the ways that the distance between a hypothetical "us" and a "them," perhaps the able and the disabled, has a particular structure. Yet we must look at the steps from other angles, along other axes.

What are the attitudes, requirements, and practices that might represent boundaries, jumps on the graph, risers on the steps? Are there chutes, or are there ladders, set up to speed movement from top to bottom or bottom to top? What forces move up and down, affecting students' progress? Should we even want to get to the top? How do students go back down the steps or out of the university gates and back to home communities? What makes this journey possible or impossible? What does it mean to skip the steps? Where do the steps actually start?

How might we chart the steps of our own ascendance or decline (perhaps on a 2-dimensional picture or a graph)? Can we recognize perspectives from the bottom? Can we be both at the top step and at the bottom step—do we straddle steps as we climb or fall? Does the perspective of teachers, having in some way climbed above the students in their classes, change the view of the steps? What aspects of higher education's labor practices (or investments) serve to solidify these steps? What is it like to be a graduate student teacher on this map, moving from one position to another, or what it is like to be an adjunct professor?

Finally, if we want to circumvent the climb, find another way in aside from the steps, how do we build a ramp?

In the next chapter, I will begin to address this question.

CHAPTER TWO

The Retrofit

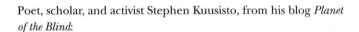

Poet, scholar, and activist Stephen Kuusisto, from his blog *Planet of the Blind*:

"Higher education administrators tend to imagine that 'someone else' will 'take care' of 'those people' who have disabilities.
American higher education still imagines that the Victorian
approach to disability is acceptable–that the disabled are taken
care of by people who will read to them in the dark." ("Higher
Education," n.p.)

As mentioned, this book is organized around three spatial metaphors.
Now that we have discussed steep steps our first metaphor, we'll move
on to explore and analyze a second one, the retrofit, characterized by
structures like ramps and curb cuts.

This chapter begins on the White House lawn, where the Americans
with Disabilities Act (ADA) was signed into law by President George Her-
bert Walker Bush over 25 years ago, in 1990. There is a famous image
that shows Bush signing the Act into being. He is flanked on either side
by disability rights activists Evan Kemp and Harold Wilke to his right,
and Sandra Parrino and Justin Dart on his left. This image takes a prominent place at the Bush Presidential Library in College Station, Texas.
In fact, the ADA and the Clean Air Act are two of the most celebrated
accomplishments memorialized in this library. Both can be seen as totally
emblematic of the retrofit. Not just because, quite technically, the Clean

Air Act and the ADA have created a huge industry out of retrofitting. But also because something like the ADA might be seen to activate the late-capitalist, neoliberal co-optation of progressive values within a token and minimalistic framework. In simpler terms, the ADA gets talked about as a huge leap in human rights, but it delivers very little. In fact, this is how it does most of its damage: it ensures that only very little gets done. Thousands of very little things like ramps get created, and this may in fact stall progress on much bigger issues.

Lennard Davis has argued that, "certainly, an ADA could not pass today" (*Enabling Acts* 8). And as historian of disability activism Mary Johnson has shown, the ADA was a "highly compromised piece of legislation," and almost immediately took "a beating in both the court of law and the court of public opinion" (127). In her words, "critics of the ADA have successfully cast people who use the law as malcontents who hurt the rest of us. Many Americans have fallen for the argument that there are 'disabled people' and 'the rest of us'—the former divided into the truly disabled (read: deserving but few) and the fakers" (Johnson, 150).[1] The ADA has followed similar patterns of "progress and retrenchment" to laws meant to promote racial equity and equality. There is progress, then there is backlash, laws are diluted or not enforced, and exclusions are maintained.

Take for example the earlier image of a young black woman crawling backward up the Capitol steps. In other pictures from this protest, a much younger girl was pictured. This young woman was Jennifer Keelan, and she was just eight years old when she got out of her wheelchair to climb the steps and take part in this protest—and had her picture taken. Jennifer was actually consulted when the ADA was written not long after the protest, and she wanted to ensure that she would be able to ride on the same bus with her sister, thus ensuring that public transit was covered. She earned an award for her contributions in 1990, when the law was passed. But when she was interviewed in 2015, 25 years later, she was struggling to find accessible housing in Colorado, and had experienced periods of homelessness. One of the authors of the ADA, Jennifer said that in reality, currently, the law was altogether too easy to avoid and ignore, adding that she was still climbing steep steps (access "The Little Girl").

For instance, although laws like the ADA are supposed to have created a much more accessible Internet, research has shown that "the way that the disability rights law currently stands allows the practices of private, non-profit, and public entities to undermine the overarching goals of the law in terms of accessible technology" (Wentz et al., n.p.). In fact, "the law encourages the creation of inaccessible information and communication technologies that may eventually become accessible, but often do not. The current state of the law allows for separate but equal, but usually results in simply unequal" (Wentz et al., n.p.). This separation brings us a long way from the promise of the ADA, and reveals that in fact disability law can often be placed directly in the way of disability justice.

In Canada, there is similar legislation, such as the Accessibility for Ontarians with Disabilities Act (AODA). While the AODA is relatively new, and is relatively untested legally, it is already invoked as a sort of specter of punishment—it is rarely mentioned without also discussing the fines that will be incurred if it is violated (up to $100,000 a day) or the "lawsuits waiting to happen." Yet there are no formal mechanisms for reporting violations—and so it continues to exist purely as a threat—while it also divides the population between disabled and nondisabled, thus constructing disabled bodies as part of this threat.

This threat seems only to be increasing (as threats generally do). As Hua Hsu wrote in the *New Yorker*, 2015 was the "year of the imaginary college student." In mainstream publications and higher educational periodicals alike "there were tales of students seeking 'trigger warnings' before being exposed to potentially upsetting class materials" among other grievances and "every week seemed to bring additional evidence for the emerging archetype of the hypersensitive college student" (n.p.). Hsu critiques these students, but also more generously suggests that "perhaps it goes both ways, and the reason that college stories have garnered so much attention this year is our general suspicion, within the real world, that the system no longer works" (n.p.). It would be worthwhile to try and apply this same suggestion, at the very least, to students with disabilities seeking accommodations, because to seek an accommodation or a trigger warning is not to ask for a special advantage within a world in which your needs are centered—rather, it is to identify your needs within a framework in which everyone (from teachers to administrators to pundits) seems to know what college students need, and who they are, better than they do themselves; a world in which any small, real adjustment can be quickly inflated into a "state of the kids these days" fictionalization; a realm in which asking for help is immediately stigmatized. It should not be difficult to imagine that accommodations for students with disabilities not only exist in a learning environment that no longer works but also that these accommodations can often increase what's broken.

The picture on the White House lawn has become canonical—but it also centers Bush Sr.'s role in this civil rights breakthrough, and White (House)-washes or Bushwhacks the actual activist history. So the memorials in the Bush Library should serve to remind us of the ways that the retrofit can be used to subsume and overwrite movements toward diversity and inclusion. Retrofits address inequities and inaccessibility, but do so in ways that reinforce ableism, turning disabled people into charity cases or villains, while situating teachers, administrators—and even presidents—as heroes.

So my second spatial metaphor—and the concept organizing this second chapter—is the retrofit. Retrofits like ramps "fix" space, but retrofits also have a chronicity—a timing and a time logic—that renders them highly temporary yet also relatively unimportant. Thus the experience of seeking a retrofit usually reveals that they are slow to come and fast to expire. Anyone who has waited for a wheelchair bus, or the key to an accessible elevator, or waited around while either of these things broke down and needed to be repaired, can identify this chronicity or timing.[2]

In my approach, I mentioned that disablism can never be fully disconnected from ableism. Academia powerfully mandates able-bodiedness and able-mindedness, as well as other forms of social and communicative hyperability, and this can best be defined as ableism. But what we also learn from higher education is that disablism is almost always wrapped into, and sometimes hidden within, ableism. Retrofits help us to understand this relationship. That is, when the accommodations that students with disabilities have access to, over and over again, are intended to simply temporarily even the playing field for them in a single class or activity, it is clear that these retrofits are not designed for people to live and thrive with a disability, but rather to temporarily make the disability go away. The aspiration here is not to empower students to achieve with disability, but to achieve around disability or against it, or in spite of it. The disablism built into that overarching desire for able-bodiedness and able-mindedness comes from the belief that disability should not and cannot be something that is positively claimed and lived-within. There is a structural ableism to the university: a way of repeatedly rewarding bodies and minds and forms of communication and sociality that are the right (constrained) shape. But there is also an explicit disablism that denigrates specific bodies and minds and forms of communication and sociality. The retrofit is one way in which we address structural ableism (for instance an inaccessible space) with means that simply highlight and accentuate and invite disablism—for instance, singling out the body that needs to ask for access.

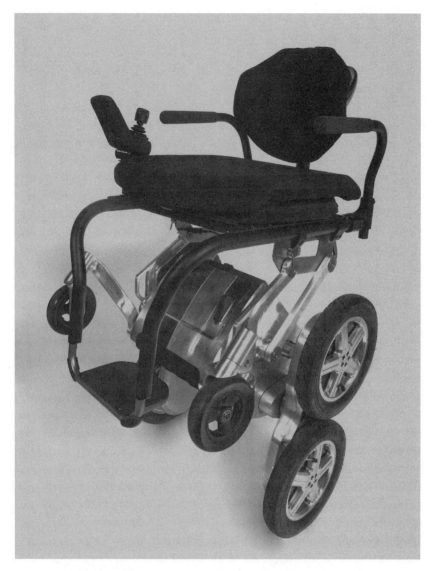

Fig. 4. The iBot Climbing Wheelchair. Toyota Corporation.

Take for example the notion (from a recent Vice article) that we should "Repair Disabilities, Not Sidewalks," or this image of the iBot Climbing Wheelchair:

The image depicts a modern black, electric wheelchair with six wheels. The four large wheels on the chair can rest on two separate steps of a set of stairs, though (very notably) there is no one in the chair. The smaller front set of swiveling wheels on the chair is up in the air. The chair appears to have a cantilevering system that would allow the individual sitting in the chair to remain upright as the chair goes down the stairs, though one would have to imagine that there would be a substantial bump each time the wheels moved down a step (access Istvan).

Inventions such as this, and the accompanying argument that it would be better to create stair-climbing wheelchairs than build ramps or elevators, or simply create level entrances to more buildings, actually distill what happens when disability is "accommodated" in higher education more clearly than the metaphor of the ramp does. A ramp, even when it is mainly used by disabled people, exists in the public sphere. But a primary message around accommodation is that disability is isolating and individuating, something located within a single and singular body. The demand is that that one body be adapted to a curriculum (or structure or terrain) that is otherwise unwelcoming, inaccessible, inhospitable to that body and mind. The climbing wheelchair may not even be very good at driving on anything but stairs; it may not be particularly safe to use on most stairs anyhow; it may be big and ugly; it likely is tremendously expensive. It is estimated that the iBot costs $25,000 US. But these are all expected outcomes and seem like reasonable problems or burdens for the individual disabled body to deal with in an ableist culture.

Moving from purely physical examples to a broader view of access, a trigger warning can also be seen as a kind of retrofit. For much more on the backlash against trigger warnings from a disability studies perspective, readers should access Angela Carter's excellent "Teaching with Trauma: Trigger Warnings, Feminism, and Disability Pedagogy." As Carter writes, "An accurate understanding of trauma and triggers situates trauma in the context of disability, not discomfort, and it illustrates the persistent misconceptions surrounding disability and mental illness" (n.p.). Further: "when faculty position themselves against trigger warnings because of justifiable fears of increased work load, expanded emotional labor, or risks of retribution, they create a false binary between one group experiencing institutional exploitation and another. The needs of faculty and staff need not be positioned against the needs of students" (n.p.). In "Weepy Rhetoric, Trigger Warnings, and the Work of Making Mental Illness Visible in the Writing Classroom," Sarah Orem and Neil Simpkins also write that "because they call attention to the emotional pain of students, trigger warnings tap into longstanding assumptions about mental illness—namely, that mentally ill persons are merely malingering, dwelling unnecessarily with emotional pain, and in need to toughening up" (n.p.). At its most simple, a trigger warning is a way to admit that abuse happens at universities. Thus, when professors and universities ban them, what they are banning is the mention of their own complicity in violence—this is an easy and a natural thing for universities to want to do. They neither want to admit that they have students in pain nor to admit that they could be the cause of that pain. Instead, professors and universities want to position themselves as working with whole students who they improve. Refusing to use trigger warnings, or using them purely as a thoughtless preface or add-on, prevents us from having a real conversation about trauma. The steep steps approach to teaching refuses the idea of trigger warnings. The retrofitted approach uses trigger warnings carelessly, simply throwing a TW on a syllabus, refusing to recognize that, as Orem and Simpkins argue, "trigger warnings frequently mark pain that is explicitly gendered or racialized, like rape or police violence[;] they perform the kind of work that . . . is forbidden by dominant systems of oppression" (n.p.). A trigger warning can save a student (or a reader of a book) from being, metaphorically, thrown down a set of stairs. But trigger warnings also need to incite a larger discussion about structural ableism and systemic violence.

All of this said, in an educational context, we will likely continue to have to work with and through the logic of the retrofit. The previous chapter on the "steep steps" should help us to recognize this. But we also need to allow for an environment in which students can claim difference without fear of discrimination and in which this claiming doesn't simply result in the student assuming all of the risk. Disability also can't be seen as something frozen in time and frozen in othered bodies—it has to be embraced as an always-everywhere, as a material but always changing reality. But we need retrofits that alter the negative impact of disability for the better, rather than preserving the stigma, the delay, and the conditional and temporary nature of access. In the classroom, we can't simply expect disabled students to strap into the ideological, pedagogical equivalent of a climbing wheelchair.

Defeat Devices

A recent controversy about Volkswagen car engines highlights the negative nature of so many retrofits and offers us a perhaps-better term: the "defeat device." These are defined as technologies that respond to or monitor engines and then regulate the emission control system to reduce its effectiveness. The devices could basically trick the emission control system so that the car might be able to pass emissions inspections, but would still, in practice, be able to emit noxious chemicals. These devices had little purpose beyond confounding the purpose of emissions controls. Likewise, many accommodations are actually designed only to meet the legal standard and actually serve to mask other forms of discrimination, prevent positive and ongoing change, and encourage teachers and administrators in their game of make-believe.

Allow me to match this with a recent anecdote. A colleague recently posted on social media that disabled students had come to them with institutional accommodation forms, but said, "Actually the way you've designed this course, there's nothing I need changed to accommodate me." Ostensibly, they had seen the syllabus and decided that the class was going to meet their needs. It sounds like a nice, feel-good story. But it actually may be evidence of the syllabus as defeat device. The relatively new practice of turning the "ask" for accommodations into in-person exchanges between students and teachers lends itself to the kind of huge power imbalance that could make a student say something like this even when it isn't true, especially if this is the type of student who wants to make a good first impression.[3] Further, just as we now know that emissions can't be effectively monitored in a single test, teaching takes place over the course of a semester and every class offers new opportunities for accommodation and for exclusion.

In a *Chronicle of Higher Education* essay published in March 2017, Gail A. Hornstein recounts a similar exchange, albeit lamenting "Why I Dread the Accommodations Talk." Her argument is that she actually knows much better than students do, or offices of Disability Services do, what accommodations a student who experiences panic attacks needs.

The major "defeat device" in teaching, then, may be our own magical thinking, or self-congratulation, or willingness to insert ourselves as more expert than students or disability officers. And I say our here intentionally: the teacher in the first scenario could easily have been me or might be me in the future. And certainly, there are readers who perhaps see themselves as the teacher in one or both of the above scenarios. But the students in the first anecdote seem to have closed off the possibility of asking for more later. They have endorsed the accessibility of the class before it has really even begun—and that assumes that we know exactly in what ways a course will be or become inaccessible before it begins. In the second scenario, the teacher moves from a perhaps-reasonable critique of the accommodations process into a move that strips the student of agency, and bypasses her rights.

In these instances, we can find many possible defeat devices in our pedagogy—and we must. But we also must interrogate the contractual moment of asking for accommodations, as well as the legalistic framework within which this exchange is governed. Sticking with the bare minimum accommodations can be dangerous, and so can assuming that we know better. Both of these responses work as defeat devices.

Dale Katherine Ireland identifies defeat devices that work as "uncanny accommodations": they seem like they should work (perhaps to the office of disability services, perhaps to the student, perhaps to the teacher), and they just don't (n.p.). [4] For instance, the single most-applied accommodation at universities is extended time to take tests and exams. Yet Laura Sokal and others have shown that there is little research showing the efficacy of this adjustment. This doesn't mean the accommodation doesn't work for some students, sometimes—it just shows that offices of disability services generally offer a very narrow range of possibilities to students, with little engineering for difference. In this climate, accommodations can be much more about being seen to do something rather than searching for the right thing. And, on the other hand, we cannot assume that teachers know best. Hornstein, for example, convinces herself that it is best for the student not to really receive any accommodations at all, and assumes that the student succeeded in her class because of this tough-love attitude, not in spite of it.

Cover Your Ass

As Jeffrey Willett and Mary Jo Deegan write, many retrofits are "far too limited in number or implementation," or are simply absurd (146). Their list of examples nicely illustrates the ways that retrofitting can preserve exclusion:

> The number of [accessible] hotel rooms and parking spaces cannot meet demands . . . accessible rooms [are provided] in largely inaccessible buildings . . . the person with a disability [may have to] travel two or three times farther to enter a building than the distance needed to use the able-bodied entrance. Ramps leading to these entrances may be the last cleared of ice and snow. Elevators may be poorly situated, slow, or too small. Many large lecture halls and movie theatres force people in wheelchairs to sit at the back. (146)

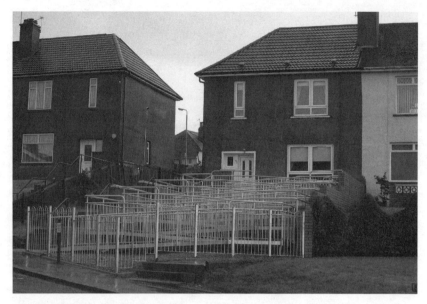

Fig. 5. "Katie Lalley's Access Ramp." Courtesy of SWNS.com.

As with the example of the "defeat device," altogether too many retrofits preserve or perpetuate exclusion rather than address it. They are about covering your ass, legally—not about creating anything like real access.

Take, for instance, this "retrofitted" ramp added to the front of public housing in Clydebank, Scotland, and think about how the retrofit physically slows the young person who requested that ramp, while foregrounding their status as a "misfit" in capitalist society, both as someone who lives in subsidized housing, and as someone subject to a disingenuous and perhaps even dangerous nod to inclusion.

The image shows a view of the concrete ramp from the sidewalk in front of a small, red-brick, semidetached house. The ramp has 10 levels—it runs diagonally from side to side 10 times. The entire ramp is enclosed on both sides by heavy gauge steel railings. Imagine: How long does it take to get up or down this ramp? How does the ramp stigmatize the family, as every other home has a small grass lawn in front, but this house has thousands of kilograms of steel and concrete? This image distills the chronology (or the timing) and the absurdity of accommodation. The idea of offering an accessible entrance to this young woman is a good one; the implementation destroys or reverses this sentiment.

This is the house of a seven-year old girl who uses a wheelchair. Her mom petitioned the council of the public housing estate for access to their house, and the response, after two years of lobbying, was this, taking up their entire yard and costing almost US$100,000. That all the articles about it mention this dollar value also helps to construct disability as a drain. But it is a terrifically depressing and perfect encapsulation of the logic of the retrofit: it took two years to get a terrible solution, one that marks their house out as a spectacle, one that will probably mean that seven year old has to spend about 30 minutes to get to her front door. The ramp makes an aesthetic statement, it is an ideology in steel—an object that has the wasting of time and the depletion of energies built into its bolts. The ramp also makes a plain statement about the ways that disability is built into the spaces and times of contemporary society. Retrofits like this are passive aggressive. In fact, passive aggression might describe the affect (or emotional life) of most retrofits. Passivity and aggression also seem to describe the timing of retrofits, as they so often aggressively delay access.

In relegating disability to the margins, retrofits serve as what might be called abeyance structures—perhaps allowing for access, but disallowing the possibility of action for change. Abeyance means to hold back, and this wheelchair ramp holds back and delays as much as it provides access. Retooling the gas engine, for example, might save gas, but it also might delay research into renewable fuel sources, or alternatives to the cult of the car.

That said, the retrofit, because it reveals what might be called an essential "supplementarity" in any culture or structure, is not wholly a bad thing. More simply, even the presence of ramps clues us in to the fact that buildings were planned and built poorly in the beginning. I am not, in fact, arguing against such accommodations. Instead, I hope to show how the presence of such temporary additions—limited in their time of effectiveness and in their space of implementation—will always point up the lack, the partiality of social and architectural structures. This lack shouldn't be either lamented or ignored, but rather addressed. The presence of retrofits cannot be seen as completing this lack, or filling in the holes.

Since the passage of the ADA in 1990, the public has begun to understand disability as an issue of space. This issue is constructed as a matter of compliance, as the dominant terminology of the act is the idea of reasonable accommodation. The "reason" of the medical and legal establishment, then, finally decides upon which accommodations are to be made. What this means in practice is that, in higher education, we witness a large industry of lawyers and HR managers and administrators paid to determine what exactly can be gotten away with under the rubric of "undue hardship" or the "undue burden" of accommodations. For instance, as Stuart Selber has shown, schools like Cornell have determined that a university website does not need to be made accessible until it is read by a certain number of people (n.p.).[5] Shockingly, when the U.S Department of Education determined that thousands of hours of video teaching materials – 20,000 course videos – hosted by U.C Berkeley were not accessible, Berkeley simply yanked down the videos from public-facing sites rather than captioning them. The clear message is that accessibility is simply not worth it. An implicit message is that the mandate for accessibility 'spoils things' for everyone else (access "Erasing"). Making all sites accessible immediately, or when they are being built, is somehow an "undue burden" and not a "reasonable accommodation"; it is also rarely, rarely done.

Yet since the ADA, at the very least, people with disabilities have been given space. The construction of elevators or ramps instead of steep steps, these are well-intentioned ideas; they speak to our desire for equality. Yet, as Patricia Sullivan has written, this democratic ideal of equality, when faced with "a broad and diverse cross-section of American culture . . . in college classrooms" can also lead the university to respond with "a humane disregard for difference under an egalitarian ethic" (39). This egalitarian ethic might be labeled fairness. As Kimber Barber-Fendley and Chris Hamel point out, however, fairness is an incredibly underdefined term. They argue that fairness is spatialized, metaphorized, as the "level playing field" (512). The retrofit—in my mind the contemporary even playing field response to disability—is a sort of cure, but halfhearted, and so it begins by negating disability and ends up only partially succeeding, thus leaving many people with disabilities in difficult positions.

The fact is, too often, we react to diversity instead of planning for it. We acknowledge that our students come from different places, and that they are headed in different directions, yet this does little to alter the vectors of our own pedagogy or teaching. Most often, the only time disability is spoken or written about in class is in the final line of the syllabus, when students are referred to Disability Services should they desire assistance.[6] The message to students is that disability is a supplementary concern—and then that it is not the teacher's concern, not really a part of the course; it's at the back door of the syllabus. The sentence about Disability Services gets the syllabus up to spec. Teachers deal with disability via the ideological equivalent of a ramp—disability as an identity category can come in the side or the back entrance, if it is to be included at all.

Like the saying "what happens in Vegas stays in Vegas," the retrofit also ensures that whatever accommodation happens in a single class stays in that class only. That is, we are encouraged, by the logic of the retrofit, to only change slightly for one student at one time, not to alter our teaching for all students in more permanent ways. Also, teachers are encouraged to view disability as something to be addressed only when it arises, never to let it extend beyond the classroom and into scholarship and service. The student must also ask for the same accommodations, chosen from a limited menu, again and again and again.

Of course, the intellectual implications of the retrofit are many. When we analyze the buildings of our universities and cities, we can understand how thought about disability has almost always been a side-thought or an afterthought: count the appended ramps, the painted-in parking spots, the stair-lifts. Their presence should not make us feel satisfied; they should call up the repeated, layered, nearly overwhelming presence of exclusive structures. To repeat myself: this should always remind us that, if rhetoric is the circulation of discourse through the body, then spaces and institutions cannot be disconnected from the bodies within them, the bodies they selectively exclude, and the bodies that actively intervene to reshape them.

So it would be useful—in society as a whole and within higher education in particular, to make clear distinctions between retrofits and defeat devices. Too many retrofits do not actually increase access. Further, we must work to decouple the presence of accommodations from the notion of access. Accommodations are accommodations: they cannot promise anything like actual, real access. Finally, when accommodations are present, we need to better understand their true emotional and physical and temporal costs.

The Affect of Accommodation

Accommodations are carried out, or otherwise anchored, by the actions of university offices of learning assistance or disability services—or more recently and more euphemistically, by AccessAbility services.[7] These offices are, first and foremost, concerned with enforcing the reasonable accommodations mandated by the ADA or other laws. The following message, used by Southern Mississippi University ODA, or Office of Disability Accommodations, describes this process:

> Students wanting to receive accommodations for a disability must complete an ODA application and provide documentation of the disability. Documentation must include a statement explaining how the disability, with or without mitigating circumstances, limits a major life area, thus impacting a student's participation in courses, programs, services, activities, and facilities. ODA does not assist students in obtaining appropriate documentation, nor does ODA refer students for eligibility evaluations. Students who do not have current documentation of a disability and who request referrals for such evaluations will be provided a resource directory of appropriate community agencies and professionals. All fees associated with procuring documentation are the responsibility of the student. (n.p.)

Clearly, another entailment of the accommodation model is the idea that it is the student him or herself who must prove that they need accommodations, and argue for them reasonably.[8] As Joe Stramondo has pointed out, in an article entitled "The Medicalization of Reasonable Accommodation," "using medical experts as the gatekeepers" is a way to avoid "fraud"—but this amounts to a "disincentive for an already marginalized group to claim what is theirs. In effect, through their medicalization, the reasonable accommodations of the ADA have, at least partially, become barriers to the inclusion of disabled people in the academy" (n.p.).

There is a clear rhetoric in this accommodation discourse as well, an attitude of indifference toward the individual, and a refusal to provide support until this support is legally mandated. Following this process, the accommodations offered still demand that the student must accommodate him or herself to the dominant logic of classroom pedagogy. Once we begin to go down the road of accommodating disability, we are also admitting that dominant pedagogies privilege those who can most easily ignore their bodies, and those whose minds work the most like the minds of their teachers (likely meaning, as well, those who look much like their teachers). And yet the keyword of the retrofit is compliance. Despite the fact that we certainly hope none of our students is holding up "compliance" as one of their key goals for their education—we hope that graduates won't just be writing "I am highly compliant" on their job letters or personal profiles postgraduation—compliance continues to be the key goal for accommodation and accessibility.

What this focus on compliance does, in the words of Stephen Kuusisto, is to turn the request for accommodation into an invitation for "gestural violence":

[P]redicated by inconvenience—a blind graduate student needs multiple streams of accessible information if she's to succeed. The Dean or Associate Dean finds this request threatening for she knows nothing about the ways and means of delivering accessible information. It's vexatious, the request, the ignoble "ask" because the system is incommodious. . . . It works by deflection. It works by assumptions. If you were a better disabled person you wouldn't be bothering me. If you were less blind you'd be easier to deal with. If only you had a better attitude about life. Gestural violence is automatic. It is invariably disgraceful, shockingly unacceptable, and yet, tied to dominance, it is widespread within higher education. ("Disability," n.p.)

Another response comes from teachers who "[find] or, if necessary [invent] an extreme example of [a disabled] student's 'demands'" ("Becoming Visible," 378). The validity or veracity of a student's claim to disability is debated by the teacher, rather than defined by the student or even by the legal and medical paradigm. Students with learning disabilities come to be seen as "jumping the queue, cutting the line, pushing patient, suffering 'average' kids out of the way and into the shadows while they, waving their label, rush to the front to grab an oversized piece of the shrinking pie" (Brueggemann et al., 378).[9]

On the other extreme, accommodation is often seen as an act of charity. Really good teachers and administrators, who really care about "them," help them to overcome themselves. Accommodation requests thus also get the "tone police" treatment—where students are encouraged to perform the role of gracious, thankful subject, to praise good professors and administrators and never complain. There is no feedback loop: if an accommodation is given, the student is expected to be fully thankful and happy, regardless of the fit of the accommodation or its efficacy. The affect of accommodation is just as tightly prescribed and prescripted as are its pedagogical or classroom parameters. Or, more simply said: students have to feel and act fully accommodated at all times, even when they are not.

So, a student becomes the object of the medical gaze, and hence the object of therapeutic and corrective pedagogy. Or the student evades this process and remains invisible. Or the student is seen as flouting disability instead of pulling herself up by the bootstraps. Or their needs are deflected and defeated. Or the academy makes (a limited range of) accommodations its moral mission, making students with disabilities objects of pity. With only these possibilities, and with these possibilities reinforcing one another, students with disabilities face a difficult terrain.

Disability support office employees and researchers Kimber Barber-Fendley and Chris Hamel have examined the rhetoric of accommodation at length. Their work is of interest as it sorts through a history of disciplinary attitudes toward learning disability. They advocate for what they call "underground" accommodations, through a program of Alternative Assistance. Such a program allows students to access accommodations somewhat secretly, in concert with teachers and disability services offices, and this mitigates some of the stigma an individual student might face in coming out in class. The program also extends across a student's university career, so that accommodations aren't just temporary patches over pedagogy. But, of course, nothing is done to confront stigmatization as a cultural problem. The message is that disability should be secret—disability must sink below the mainstream; surface pedagogy-as-usual is not disturbed. Disability is alternative to classroom culture. What the authors don't mention in their article is that the program they refer to and advocate for, through the Strategic Alternative Learning Technologies center at the University of Arizona, costs students $2,100 per semester, on top of the cost of securing documentation of their disability, and of course normal tuition. The price tag reveals another problem: being non-normal costs the individual. Across North America, the cost of disability is a controversial issue—many schools want to dissuade students with disabilities from applying and enrolling, because it is believed that their needs cost more. As Rod Michalko and Tanya Titchkosky point out, "the presence of disabled students at a university represents, for some, the requirement of additional expense . . . a drain upon university resources" ("Putting Disability in Its Place," 219). Illegal and unconscionable as it is, this market is allowed to discipline the student body, effecting restraints and implanting normative self-regulations in student, teacher, and institution, concurrently implementing or sustaining, or both, the same logics in society. More simply, all other students cost money to educate as well, of course—and most of them also pay tuition. But students with disabilities are (in general) the only ones who are uniquely constructed economically—they cost too much. Other students are seen as investments to be protected. Yet campus policies are generally designed to protect the university from disabled students—as physical threats, as threats to the intellectual freedom of educators, as lawsuit threats, as always-already cheating the system.

For example, recently disgraced Mount St. Mary's University (Maryland) president Simon Newman publicly discussed a plan to find out which first-year students might be suffering from depression and kick these students out before they could impact the university's retention rates. Infamously, he likened these students to bunnies that didn't need to be cuddled. Instead, he told faculty, "You just have to drown the bunnies . . . put a Glock to their heads" (Young Lee). Newman, however, felt he was just running the university like a good business. If funding relied on having better retention numbers, and he estimated that forcing 20–25 students out immediately would increase these numbers by 4–5 percent, then that was what needed to be done. As rhetoric and writing scholar Pegeen Reichert Powell argues, citing earlier work on retrofitting, "retention efforts are a kind of retrofit that, like basic-writing courses or ramps for people with physical disabilities, treat failure as the problem of the individual rather than that of the institution" (98). This is just one of the by-products of the "good business" of academic administration.

This managerial rhetoric is unsurprising. It is part of a well-noticed, well-understood trend. More and more often, we see chief executive officers (like Newman) hired away from the private sector to run colleges and universities, even large research schools. This replaces the general trend of having academia "self-governed" by academics, even at the presidential level. Of course, in analyzing *The Emergence of the American University* at the turn of the 20th century, Laurence Veysey pointed out that even at that time there were two types of academics: those who insulated themselves from the public and even from students in order to perform research, and those "administrators who might almost as easily have promoted any other sort of American enterprise," and knew how to run and talk about higher education as a business with American values (443). More recently, we would suggest that academics have what Donna Strickland calls a "managerial unconscious"—one that syncs up with the demand for white collar workers. So, whether unconsciously implanted in the minds of academic administrators, or overt in the words and deeds of the chief executive officer administrators imported into academia, this business model has specifically dangerous ways to respond to and to construct disability.

As more colleges and universities are run like businesses, and as governments continue to defund schools so that they need to rely more and more on private funding, which increases this orientation to a business model, we can expect that disability will continue to be constructed as a drain, a threat, something to be eradicated or erased—not worth retaining.

From Eradication to Negotiation

The normative demand in academia is that disability must disappear. Accommodation rhetoric echoes this demand in slightly less loud, but equally insistent, tones. A disability studies perspective asks us to think about how what we do enables and disables, once we allow that disability exists. Inclusion should mean the presence of significant difference— difference that rhetorically reconstructs—though often people with disabilities have such change-agency qualified or revoked. Gerard Goggin and Christopher Newell interrogate the rhetoric of inclusion as it frames technological issues for people with disabilities:

> People with disabilities are expected to cut their cloth to fit the temporarily able-bodied world, and its new media technologies. Paradoxically, in its desire for the same, inclusion always requires the "other" to stay in its niche as it is pressed into the mold of the normal, rather than engaging with the real alterity and difference in an "us" relationship. (149)

 Inclusion can be used as a panacea, a word that might register the presence of difference, while keeping its participation delayed. Patricia Dunn has also argued that, "total immersion in the mainstream [for students with disabilities], while not altering the mainstream, will not work" (115). Cynthia Lewiecki-Wilson has suggested that people with disabilities often find themselves "arguing, or being pushed towards the argument, 'we just want to be treated like everyone else,'" thereby diluting the transformative potential of their participation in the public forum" ("Re-Thinking," 159). The perspective of disability, then, shouldn't just be included in the classroom, shouldn't just be reflected in the design of our teaching practices and technologies; it must change what we do.

I want to suggest that, in some cases, a retrofitting can be useful, can aid students in their navigation of this space—just as an elevator or a ramp might enable mobility. But we need a more sophisticated form of negotiation in order to retrofit structures and practices in the best possible way. We need to think through the academic spaces that we inhabit and build and the bodies that are written and ruled by—and that rewrite—these spaces. With the above-mentioned attitudes toward disability, negotiation is rarely evident. Instead, people with and (supposedly) without disabilities are forced to work around an inaccessible environment, never cooperating because too often their concerns are perceived as divergent (or in competition). We need to allow for an environment in which students can claim difference without fear of discrimination. This environment must include disability—currently, it rarely does. Further, disability cannot be seen as something one person diagnoses in another. Disability must be seen as socially negotiated; people with disabilities must be seen as the moderators, the agents of this negotiation.

In "Disability Geography," Deborah Metzel and Pamela Walker emphasize the importance of negotiative roles for people with disabilities. The authors write that "in deliberate contrast to traditional service models [for people with disabilities] . . . individualized approaches are designed to enhance community presence and participation" (127). This individualized negotiation would expand "social-spatial lives of people with disabilities and [promote] increased control and spatial choice" (127). John Dewey, in *Experience and Education*, quite clearly emphasizes the importance of negotiation. He writes that "the principle of interaction makes it clear that failure of adaptation of material to needs and capacities of individuals may cause an experience to be non-educative quite as much as a failure of an individual to adapt himself to the material" (47). For Dewey, this represents "a failure in education, a failure to learn one of the most important lessons of life, that of mutual accommodation and adaptation" (68). For Dewey, this adaptation was to be ongoing—he united interaction and situation as his key concepts of education when he wrote about this topic back in the 1930s (41). Simply, there could be no set materials and methods—instead of viewing set approaches to set groups of students as intentional and rational, he foregrounded the role of changing environments, the context of a community, the wide diversity of learners, and argued that "lack of mutual accommodation [makes] the process of teaching and learning accidental" (45). Dewey's is a difficult position to argue for in an era of standardized testing and "no child left behind" curriculum. The position that intentional, clinical, standardized education would be only accidentally successful, and that only co-intentional and situated education could be malleable enough for success is hard to make nowadays. Yet without something like this shift, we will continue to have accidental success for some students, anchored in the structural exclusion of others. This structural exclusion will be abetted and allowed by forms of temporary, tokenized, and tenuous inclusion.

Digital Curb Cuts (to Nowhere)

One of the most prominent examples of the retrofit has always been the curb cut—dips incorporated or cut into the sidewalk so that wheelchairs can roll up rather than needing to be lifted over this lip. These cuts eventually allowed others to more easily move around—with strollers, on skateboards and bikes, and so on. Back in 1999, Steve Jacobs wrote about the "Electronic Curb-Cut Effect," showing that "unusual things happen when products are designed to be accessible to people with disabilities. It wasn't long after sidewalks were redesigned to accommodate wheelchair users that the benefits of curb cuts began to be realized by everyone" (n.p.). His argument was that Section 255 of the Telecommunications Act of 1996 could and should be used to create digital or electronic curb cuts for all. As Cynthia Waddell has written, Section 255 "was the first product design law to attempt to drive the market to create accessible products. It is not a traditional civil rights law since it is an accessible design law that does not depend on the filing of a complaint for its requirements to be enforced" (342). Jacobs created a long list, with links, of the technologies that were originally developed for people with disabilities but now benefit all: from the first typewriter, created in 1808 for a blind woman, to 1972 when Julia Child's cooking show became the first nationally broadcast open-captioned program and Vinton Cerf developed e-mail within ARPANET, in part because he was hard of hearing and used a kind of early e-mail to communicate with his Deaf wife. We could add recent examples like Optical Character Recognition, revolutionized by Ray Kurzweil to create a reading machine for blind people. This progress then quickly led to scanners, online research databases from *Lexis Nexis* to *Google Books*, and now a million smartphone apps allowing people to translate foreign-language signs, solve equations by taking pictures of them, and on and on. Put together speech recognition and OCR, and smart phones can be seen as terrific assistive devices for people with disabilities—but we also start to view these "assistive" features as the keys to almost everything a smart phone does. Goggin and Newell have looked at the history of cell phones, suggesting that "disability has played a crucial yet overlooked role" in the development of the technology" (155). As Sara Hendren and Caitlyn Lynch argue, "all technology is assistive technology" (n.p.). Or, as Rosemarie Garland-Thomson puts it, the smartphone

> will read messages and information out loud to you whether you are
> blind or sighted. It will produce words on the screen from your voice
> whether you can use a keyboard or not. It will show you pictures of

people communicating through voices or with sign language. It will allow you to adjust the size of your text regardless of your eyesight. It will allow you to swipe a variety of touch commands with a single finger no matter how many fingers you have. . . . while smart technologies such as Siri might seem like just a lot of fun to some people, they contribute to a more democratic society—something of enormous value to us all. ("Siri," n.p.)

As Graham Pullin writes, "this challenges the so-called trickle-down effect whereby advances in mainstream design are expected to find their way into specialist products for people with disabilities, smaller markets that could not have supported their development" (xiii). Instead, things created for these smaller markets become useful—terrifically, unforeseeably useful—for all. For Pullin, or Garland-Thomson, or Hendren and Lynch, all of this provides evidence of the value of disability in design. Katie Ellis and Gerard Goggin also write about even more recent developments such as locative media technologies designed by and for people with disabilities—and how what begins as an accommodation broadly shapes social practices (272).

But, there are other trickle-down or trickle-in effects. Once many of these technologies are championed as being good for all, or once the advocacy and the politicized arguments that drove the creation of many of these technologies have drifted away, these same innovations can lose their efficacy. For instance, Sean Zdenek shows how most captions are based on a "correspondence model" wherein they "merely duplicate the soundtrack" yet miss much of the rhetorical richness of the action on screen (232). This incomplete model may be fine for those who like to have captions sometimes when they watch sports in a noisy bar, for instance. But it doesn't cut it for those who truly rely on captioning every day.

This idea of an accommodation "not cutting it" might lead us to memes of "curb cuts to nowhere"—images, posted online, of ramps and curb cuts that literally lead nowhere. There are Facebook groups devoted to images of these redundant or useless ramps and curb cuts and a Google image search returns hundreds of results. One such example comes from Massey University in New Zealand, posted by an organization called Accessibility New Zealand. Here I will reproduce not the image, but their description of the image and commentary on it:

The road is significantly lower than the building's level—nearly 2 meters. There is a lawn area around the building, with a sharp incline leading down to the road. A path was built from the building to the road, with steps. A few months ago, the steps area was redone, with a cement brick retaining wall on each side of the steps, and a curb cut onto the road. There are no sidewalks by the road on either side of the stairs. While sidewalks would be safer for pedestrians currently forced to use the road, because of the retaining walls, putting sidewalks would be difficult at best. So we end up with a curb cut leading to steps. Completely useless. It almost seems to me to be a case of "let's put a curb cut because the regulations call for them." Mindless application of the standards, with little or no thinking. (n.p.)

As an example of an outcome of a (perhaps well-meaning) interest convergence, here we have a curb cut that very well may be nice for ambulatory pedestrians, but those folks can also likely (for now) walk up that set of stairs and navigate the path through the grass at the top of them. These are a physical manifestation of a poorly written caption, a podcast without a transcript (another of Zdenek's areas of research), or a website for a disability services office that also has no alt text for the images it uses.

Consider, alongside this physical structure, another digital analogue: as Melissa Helquist has powerfully shown (and demonstrated), the ways that a screen reader moves through an inaccessible webpage can be terrifically frustrating for a user—and terrifically time consuming, with the user needing to jump back and forth through an audio file to get the information they need. Likewise, alt text for key information like charts and graphs within scientific articles very rarely offer anything but a basic title for the table, but no description at all (Helquist). So, blind or low-vision readers either do not have access to the information others are given, or they have to take very roundabout routes to get it, on a page-by-page basis.

The same rule generally applies for things like audio descriptions of films (when someone is describing the visual action on the screen). As Catherine Kudlick and Susan Schweik argue, "like the captions provided for deaf and hard-of-hearing people, the usual 'service' approach to audio description takes an existing production and overdubs a description for blind people. Most typically think of it as an access practice, an access aid that discreetly inserts information so that a blind person can enjoy visual media along with sighted family and friends" (n.p.). But it also isolates "all blind people in an audience in a group" and "this almost clinical approach to description may have come from the history of rehab and other services for the blind; if description helps blind people get schooled, get jobs, good. But if it is about having fun or blind people questioning what is being presented to them or taking a lead . . ." (n.p.). In the classroom, the law dictates that we need to describe visual content on slides or video; but we also take a clinical approach to this practice (or we outsource it) instead of recognizing that careful, thick description of visual content would be great teaching for all students; or that if we shared this work or made it more responsive to the questions and needs of students, it would become even better teaching.

As mentioned, the "curb cut to nowhere" images have commonly been posted as a form of backlash against accommodations. The message is: Hey, look at how silly this fad of "architectural correctness" is. Yet the images also accurately reflect an absurdist critique of the late capitalist industry of retrofitting, or they show how most accessible design is facile, or so long as it begins addressing an inequity, or looks as though it is addressing an inequity, that is enough. The accessibility "fix" is unsatisfactory, clashes with the other messages of the space, and in fact ruins or invalidates the architectural character of the building. Disability itself is clearly "misfit" by the ableist or "normate template" that the campus was built upon (access Hamraie, n.p.). The same thing happens with alt text and with visual description in the examples above. We create digital curb cuts and ramps that lead nowhere just as readily as we create concrete ones.

#AcademicAbleism

This said, curb cuts to nowhere, and other memes of accessibility-gone-wrong, themselves can become a way to circulate antiableist critique. Thus, the curb cuts and the absurd ramps could be added to other recent online movements intended to call out colleges and universities for their inaccessibility or for the ways that their existing accommodation processes are insufficient or absurd retrofits.

Curb cuts to nowhere often depict incompletely or absurdly retrofitted academic spaces—as in the example discussed above from Clydebank University. So let me end this section by suggesting that the retrofits, curb cuts, interest convergences, and other forces and structures that make the world an ableist landscape digitally and concretely also provide us opportunities to mobilize and connect (often using digital tools). For example, the #academicableism hashtag was originally created by @zaranosaur on March 20, 2014, as a way to protest the *Guardian* (UK) newspaper's coverage of the mental health "survival strategies" of graduate students—implying that individual students needed to work harder to accommodate themselves to academic life. The hashtag has had a terrifically long life, and has created a network and community of students and faculty, exposing much of the hypocrisy around, discrimination toward, and debasement of disability within higher education.

For most students who seek accommodations for our classes, they aren't allowed to know what the actual range of accommodations might be. Instead, they have to go in to Disability Services, offer up their diagnosis, and have that diagnosis matched with a stock set of accommodations. This foregrounding of diagnosis gets at what Ellen Samuels calls the "biocertification" of disability—a "fantasy of identification" that follows from a belief that something like disability is fixed and verifiable and scientifically visible (9). The fantasy also entails that disability is not verifiable in any other way—it is a purely biological fact and viewed best (or perhaps only) by a medical professional. Yet the fantasy also allows the scientific basis of disability to be bent toward other, more subjective language and processes. As long as the biocertification is foregrounded, the process can then devolve into something much less rigid. So, in other exchanges, students might be asked by disability services to "tell us what you need"—and again students have to guess.

A student once summarized the accommodation process as being like the game *Battleship*—you can't perceive what's on the other side of the board, because there is a barrier there, and so you have to just keep trying to guess where the other player's ships are—or where the relevant accommodations are, if they exist. You throw your diagnosis over, and hope that it will land on something that will actually help you. But you cannot sense the full range of what may be on the other side, and thus you cannot directly ask for what you need.

The war metaphor may be overwrought, but at the very least students are put in the position of moving across metaphorical borders, borders that may often feel hostile. So students tell horror stories of a professor ripping up an accommodation letter, or we read of teachers citing academic freedom in refusing to provide them. When Memorial University professor Ranee Panjabi refused to wear an FM transmitter for a hard-of-hearing student, the story made national news in Canada. But other students then came out to say that Panjabi had similarly refused their accommodations requests up to 20 years previously, and the University had continued to protect the teacher while failing to enforce the accommodations ("Hard-of-Hearing"). Other teachers, in banning laptop use in their classes, force students for whom the use of a laptop is an accommodation to be clearly singled out. We have a long way to go when the very simplest of classroom accommodations become standoffs with professors pitting their own academic freedom against the needs of their students, as though the two things cannot both be safeguarded and respected.

From another angle, at times, in making the game of *Battleship* almost comically simple, offices of disability services offer a very narrow range of accommodations. As Laura Sokal recently showed, "extended testing time accommodation (ETTA) is the most common accommodation assigned to post-secondary students with disabilities," offering "150% of the standard testing time provided to other students . . . was typically assigned in over 70% of cases—despite there being no valid empirical evidence to support this practice . . . and in over 40% of these institutions there were no procedures in place for monitoring and modifying ETTA allowances once assigned" (28). What we get, then, are blanket or rubber-stamp accommodations, one size fits all—and yet even these accommodations must be asked for, over and over again, by students who are forced to hold their hand out for something that we cannot even prove helps them. As teachers, one way to defuse this "game" is to work to expand the repertoire of accommodations—every time we get an accommodation request, honor that request but also implement another appropriate one not just for that student, but for any student in a class like yours. If the accommodation that gets suggested for a student in your class doesn't fit your pedagogy, as when extended testing time is suggested but you don't give any tests, suggest something else. For example, access the accommodation "addendum" example created by Tara Wood, Melissa Helquist, and myself (Wood et al.)

Another way to think about the retrofitted accommodation is to picture the game Whack-a-Mole. Whack-a-Mole is a carnival game in which the player has a hammer. In front of the player, there is a table full of holes. The object of the game is to literally whack the small furry animatronic moles that pop up in the holes in front of us. Well, disability has become the Whack-a-Mole of higher education. When disability pops up, we slap it with a quick accommodation, and we just hope it doesn't pop up again. The nature of the "retrofitted" accommodation requires that we make no lasting changes to our pedagogy or to the culture of the university. Just whack it whenever it pops up.

For instance, walk into any faculty mailroom in the beginning of a semester, and look for the envelopes from "disability services." It is like a lottery of sorts—not having a letter in the mailbox signals that disability will not be a concern that semester. You win! The envelope encloses disability, not just in the template of the letter inside it, but also within the performative or contractual act of even opening the envelope (perhaps that's why many teachers put off taking the envelopes out of their boxes for so long, as though to delay the fact that they have a student with a disability in their class—look for this and you will notice faculty removing all other mail and delaying taking the envelopes out). Further, not having an envelope in your mailbox encourages you to not import or carry-forward past strategies you may have developed for accommodating students, and not to develop new ones. The teacher imagines a(n immediate) future without disability, and I would suggest that this (distressingly) most often feels like a relief.

At many schools now, the process of distributing the letters to teachers has been outsourced to the student themselves, as a gesture to a kind of "self-efficacy" that seems pedagogical and intentional. It's a paternalistic message to the student that they need to take control of their own accommodations, but the power differential between students and teachers is huge. If approximately two-thirds of U.S. college students with disabilities won't disclose these disabilities to seek help, they certainly won't do so if this disclosure now gets forced and repeated at the beginning of every class.

In an autoethnography (or a careful personal story, framed within cultural factors) of the collaboration between students and teachers to find accommodations, a student wrote that such

> self-advocacy is easy to preach but is another barrier in practice. Professors, who may have a bias or just indifference toward accommodations, can be a challenge for any person. I'm constantly aware that asking for an accommodation is asking professors to make an extra effort when preparing their lessons. If a professor doesn't do the accommodation, or the accommodation doesn't work, I'm timid to go back unless the lines of communication are open. I feel like Oliver Twist asking, "Please, Sir, may I have some more?" I don't want to get out of an assignment, or to have an added advantage. I've been afraid to go back to a professor because I worried my grade could be affected. (Aguirre and Duncan, 535)

The affective or emotional cost of this repeated process is obvious, as are the tangible risks.

As Laurence Veysey wrote in his canonical *The Emergence of the American University*, the patriarchal character of mid-19th-century schools created a "phenomenon known to authoritarian regimes: constant desire for a confession of guilt, and the resulting submission of will by one's inferiors" (35). There is certainly a hint of this desire in the rigid choreography of the current accommodation process, even if this strict control (perhaps) no longer effectively describes the university as a whole. And yet in the evolution of the university away from regimes of strict moral and religious control, the moments in which the school handles its students paternalistically come into sharper contrast. Confession and submission become more of a spectacle.

The envelopes involved in this process of seeking accommodations also envelop the student within them—foreclosing and sealing off other potentials and possibilities not related to the legalistic and medical discourse of the letter. This doesn't have to be a bad thing: disability identity should be an asset in many ways. Yet I would argue that it often actually is a bad thing. In locations steeped in academic ableism, accommodations are much more likely to isolate demands for change with individual students, take the form of defeat devices, and most notably to stigmatize the student and the disability. Thus it is likely true that retrofits, in other contexts, can be much more useful and powerful than they can be in higher education, mainly because of the persistence of academic ableism.

I have mentioned the "wearing out" of the experience of seeking accommodations, something Annika Konrad calls "access fatigue." In opposition to this, Konrad urges us to think through what Mia Mingus calls "access intimacy": "that elusive, hard to describe feeling when someone else 'gets' your access needs. . . . access intimacy is also the intimacy I feel with many other disabled and sick people who have an automatic understanding of access needs out of our shared similar lived experience of the many different ways ableism manifests in our lives" (n.p.). Unfortunately, such moments of connection are hard to come by for students, and are often fleeting or created only under ideal circumstances.

When disability is seen as something "suffered" by a very few, and otherwise invisible and nonpresent, then disability can never change the culture of higher education, and higher education will continue to wear out students with disabilities, to hold disability itself in abeyance, and to create access fatigue. So, here is a provocative and pessimistic question: What if the college or university is the key space, the key economic mechanism, where disability is delayed, discouraged, and diverted from changing the world?

As Jennifer Doyle has written about Title IX, the U.S. legislation that mandates gender equality, it "shapes the university's experience of its own vulnerability. A university that obeys the law is 'compliant'; a university that does not is 'non-compliant.' . . . Title IX is the administrative structure through which the university knows what exposure feels like, what vulnerability is" (Doyle, 24). I would suggest that the AODA and the ADA function in a very similar but very different way, laying the university's commitments and philosophies bare to litigation just as much as its practices and processes and structures. Doyle goes on to suggest that "the idea of Title IX has intense rhetorical effects: it gives body to an affective economy" (Doyle, 31). So do the ADA and the AODA and other legalistic, managed, administration-facing laws: but the big problem comes when we realize that "these processes introduce to us another layer of [vulnerability and possible] betrayal—one hard-wired and systemic, one in which we are betrayed by our own affective investments in an ideological apparatus like 'school'" (Doyle, 35). In this arrangement, the professor is rendered complicit in the project of ableism and betrayed by that complicity; and on the other hand impacted by this academic ableism in all of the ways they are least able to defuse its impacts. Ableism is the process by which academia reaches the pinnacle of its investments by eating itself. "Good teaching" is never as simple as choosing what educational values you hold or convey; the system is far too big for agentive choice to cancel the impact of ableism. And the processes by which students and teachers hold on within the system are very rarely the processes by which the system might be dismantled. "University resources—time, energy, thought and compassion—are absorbed by a managerial world averse to the interpersonal, to the lateral and dynamic work of education." The latter is full of risk, Doyle argues, before succinctly stating that "the classroom is the university's soft flesh" (Doyle, 112). In contrast, the logic of the retrofit is efficient and hard and angular and edged; it is gleaming metal in a neat package. Much more simply: battling academic ableism will be as difficult, messy, ongoing, bottom-up, and unpredictable as retrofitting is limited, bordered, constrained, top-down, and rubber-stamped. This said, while retrofits are something given to students to close down other possibilities, addressing academic ableism might be most effectively done by following students.

"A Rights-Demanding Bunch"

The #academicableism movement is just one sign of the growing power of student protest. A York University (Canada) student, Navi Dhanota, recently filed a human rights complaint against the school. In 2015, the Ontario Human Rights Commission intervened and the sides settled, with York agreeing to rewrite their guidelines for academic accommodation. Basically, Dhanota argued that while students might still be forced to provide medical documentation of disability, this documentation should not need to include a diagnosis. That part of the documentation can be removed—or at least students should have the right to choose to have the actual diagnosis removed. In particular, some psychological diagnoses that are highly stigmatizing would likely lead to bias and mistreatment on college campuses. As I will explore later in the book, this protection from forced disclosure can matter especially for students of color. Dhanota won the case, as mentioned, and this ruling has led to a ripple effect, at least in Canada.

In a *Toronto Star* article following this news, columnist Heather Mallick responded to these new documentation guidelines for accommodating students with mental health disabilities in Ontario's universities and colleges, kicking off the backlash. Mallick argued that these students should not only have to deal with ableism, with inaccessible physical spaces, with the lack of counseling and the surplus of stress inherent on campus, but also should be responsible for changing this culture by wearing their labeled diagnoses proudly, that they should somehow all become advocates. You won't be stigmatized, she argued; you won't have your diagnosis questioned or belittled; you won't be accused of asking for special privileges. Yet her article went on to belittle and question these diagnoses, providing perfect evidence that stigma still exists in society and that this stigma is particularly pronounced on our campuses.

She was, however, correct about one thing: "students are a rights-demanding bunch" (n.p.).

As mentioned, the new guidelines in Ontario only mean that students will no longer have to disclose their Diagnostic and Statistical Manual (DSM) diagnosis to register for mental health accommodations and supports. They still have to provide proof of disability, verified by a doctor. This means that although "biocertification" is challenged, it isn't replaced (access Samuels). Students also have the choice to disclose more specifically if they want to. But in some cases a specific diagnosis is simply not needed. The focus can be on the accommodations rather than on labels.

Yet Mallick alluded to a "rising tide" of students with disabilities on campus. The statistics paint a very different picture, as I have already noted. Twenty-seven percent of all Canadians have university degrees. But only 17.6 percent of Canadians with "mild or moderate" disabilities have postsecondary degrees (Statistics Canada). Mallick wrote that York University had only a handful of students with mental health disabilities in the past, but had 1,200 such students registered with Counselling and Disability Services last year, alluding to some sort of a fad. York has more than 40,000 students. In the general population, 13.7 percent of Canadians have a disability, and 4.4 percent of people between 15 and 24 years old have disabilities (Statistics Canada). Moreover, according to the Canadian Mental Health Association, one in five Canadians will experience a mental illness in their lifetime. At one point, Mallick used the word "scam" to suggest that students might fake a disability. But it is more realistic to assume that many disabled students are not seeking any accommodations at all. Just 1,200 students at one very large school is not a "rising tide." Instead, it might be evidence of a big hole. According to the numbers I've listed in this book, somewhere between 500 and 6,000 students at York have disabilities and are not seeking accommodations at all. Hopefully, Dhanota's case makes it possible for more of these students to seek help, and to be protected when doing so.

So what prevents disabled students from getting the supports they need and to which they have a right? There is the very stigma that Mallick reinforces in her article. This begins with the idea that the university is the space for society's most able, physically, mentally, and otherwise—not a place to admit to any weakness or challenge. There is also the quite reasonable feeling that you will be accused of faking it, even though the financial cost and labor involved in faking a disability would vastly outweigh any benefits. And the benefits are negligible—note-taking and extra time or space for tests or exams can help, but the accommodations model too often assumes that learning only happens in lectures and high-stakes tests, and hasn't kept up with the modern classroom. If, as Mallick suggests, students and teachers are on an "intellectual mission" together, then students with disabilities are being given very few provisions for this journey. As mentioned, in Canada, there are barely more than 200 professionals employed to provide disability accommodations at colleges and universities (Fichten et al.). We can assume that the stigma increases and the provisions diminish even further for Canada's nearly 200,000 graduate students. For instance, recent research shows that half of Ontario universities do not even have an accommodation policy for these students (Rose). Schools don't want more students who need accommodations, because then they would need to properly invest in support.

Yes, Mallick is quite correct in that "students are a rights-demanding bunch." Students like Navi Dhanota (or @zaranosaur) know exactly what they are asking for: privacy and equal access to education. Students often have to disclose disability in dozens of ways every day—they deserve some control over the power imbalance this involves. They are asking for these things because stigmatization is very much alive on college and university campuses; because funding for supports for students with disabilities are scarce; because reporters like Mallick continue to question their rights and suggests they are "scamming;" because postsecondary educational environments are often disabling. Students like Navi Dhanota know all of this because they also understand academic fields like Disability Studies and the history of the disability rights movement, and because they are pushing its next frontier. Dhanota is now pursuing a graduate degree in disability studies. These students are not saying "me, me, me"—they are instead very aware that those in power, like Mallick, will attempt to divide disabled students as they also doubt and downplay disability rights. As a society, we should feel that an increase in students with disabilities, and an increase in resources for these students, would be cause for celebration; that this would signal real progress.

Progress is possible, after all. Read the marketing materials of my school, or your own, and you'll read a lot about entrepreneurship, innovation, a rapidly changing "knowledge economy." Schools are reconstructing themselves, rhetorically, as nimble and responsive and disruptive. So we know that at least on the surface, they value change. In the next chapter, I will examine some of the ways higher education seeks to change its pedagogical or teaching commitments, and how disability gets figured into this innovation and progress.

Laws = process of retrofitting—
i.e. responsblize the student
& produce avoidance beh.
in teachers — reprod.
ableism

CHAPTER THREE

Imaginary College Students

―――――∾∾―――――

Malcolm Harris, writing about the true forces for educational change, in 2016:

"Capitalists will constantly seek to reshape schooling because their labor supply can always be more efficient." (n.p.)

Multimodality. Multiliteracies. These concepts have been championed in recent scholarship in my own discipline of composition, but also across the humanities, with extraordinary volume and enthusiasm. In this chapter, I will examine this push as one specific trend signaling progress in higher education, yet reproducing old exclusions. This exploration is first of all about how universities argue for change through the invention of specific types of student mind and body. This exploration is also a sort of test case: Is it possible to ever argue for educational change without reinforcing the stigma of disability?

To keep things simple, in this chapter I will define multimodality as the engagement with many modes of meaning-making. Multimodality is communication and composition across textual, linguistic, spatial, aural, and visual resources. Multiliteracies, on the other hand, is a term coined specifically by one group (the New London Group) to talk about the skill developed by communicating across these modes and the skill needed in order to communicate across these modes. Multimodality should be an agnostic, descriptive term; multiliteracy is the term that is supposed to work as an assessment, a measure. But in a way, the distinction between the terms is irrelevant because, as you will read, the terms are rarely invoked to simply describe what a student or a classroom is doing. Much more often, the terms are used interchangeably to count or diagnose or prescribe modes or literacies.[1]

So, while the arguments that support these concepts of multiplicity are ambitious, democratic, often incisively careful and critical, and hopeful, this energy does not always lead to inclusive classroom practice. Many students who think and express themselves in nonnormative ways are actually further excluded by pedagogies of multiplicity. In this way, it is imperative to understand the context of a push toward these multiples.

To begin with, disability and literacy have generally been severed by science and by law. As disability and education researchers Christopher Kliewer, Douglas Biklen, and Christi Kasa-Hendrickson show, "restricted literacy among people with disabilities has become institutionalized as a presumably natural manifestation of organic defects thought to objectively exist well beyond the reach of social, cultural, or historical consideration" (164). Authorities from doctors to immigration agents used literacy tests to establish baselines of deviancy. Kate Vieira writes that literacy is a "navigational technology that opens up some paths and closes off others, that orients and disorients, that routes and often reroutes. . . . it is also an infrastructure that regulates movement" (30, italics mine). This metaphor of literacy as mobility (and orientation) is of utmost importance to the intersections between literacy and ability, illiteracy and disability. Literacy has been used to tightly control the movement and rights of disabled people for centuries; this deeply affects what literacy is and what it can do for anyone.

As notions of literacy developed from the idea of illiteracy, so too has ability been developed only as disability has been (often arbitrarily) marked out. I allude here to the fact that the concept of "literacy" in its contemporary sense came into use only in the late nineteenth century. Previously, to be literate meant to be familiar with literature. Original definitions of literacy were based on one's ability to read the Bible or sign one's name. In this way, literacy only came about as a result of the judgment of illiteracy (access Kendall). As Karl Marx and Foucault can be seen to argue, and as disability geographer Brendan Gleeson also reminds us, the factory "produced physical disability on an industrial scale" (109). Before industrialization, though there were ideas of ability and disability, society did not comprehensively sort its citizens using disability as a criteria. Concurrently, and consequently, illiteracy has been a way to sort society, determining who can immigrate, deciding who can vote, determining the divisions of the labor force, and so on. This sorting has always been clearly biased—for instance, at Ellis Island, Russian Jews were not allowed to take literacy tests in Hebrew. Why? Because U.S. immigration restrictionists wanted to be sure that many of them would fail, and thus forced them to take the tests in Russian (access Dolmage, "Disabled upon Arrival"). In the South, literacy tests to determine who could vote were almost comedically difficult (Onion). They were designed to disenfranchise African Americans.

Like literacy, ability is defined by its inverse. It gains shape only when a negative prefix is appended, and without this prefix it has little to no social power. The concepts of disability and illiteracy might be seen to have developed in similar ways, at similar times, in the Western world, the prefixes being used with particular, and similar (perhaps connected), ends in mind. In this chapter, I will explore how, through the push for new and multiple forms of literacy, we also come to tell stories and create maps of disability.

Somnolent Samantha

Against this backdrop of illiteracy and disability, there is also a push for new forms of literacy and ability. This can be understood as a hallmark of neoliberalism: the redefinition of intellectual values that highlight the need of the individual student (or worker) to become a more flexible (and thus fungible or disposable) producer and consumer.

The rhetorical push for multimodality and multiliteracies, such as that provided by the New London Group (Cope and Kalantzis) is now more than 15 years old, but still building momentum. Behind much of the New London Group's work is the implicit argument that, in each individual learner, the more modes engaged, the better. Of course we do not all have the same proclivity, desire, or ability to develop all of our modal or literate engagements. It seems useful and pragmatic to encourage the multiple engagement of senses and learning pathways, across multiple modes, but not to map them and add them up toward a multimodal IQ. This said, Gunther Kress of the New London Group also argues that, because a culture selects and privileges certain forms of embodied engagement, some will be "affectively and cognitively at an advantage over those whose preferred sensory modes are not valued or are suppressed in their culture" (187). So it is important to remain critical not just of which literacies and modes a culture privileges but also which combinations of literacies and modes, and which interactions between literacies and modes, come to enable or disable learners in pedagogical design, in the classroom. So this chapter will help us to further attend to how disability and illiteracy come together and create one another.

Earlier, I discussed the notion that 2015 was the "year of the imaginary college student" (Hsu). I am going to extend this to suggest that there are two specific imaginary characters created by discourse about multimodality and multiliteracy, and I am going to suggest that these two characters—both of them students—link to two dominant discourses about disability in education. I'll note that these two students should bear some ironic relationship to Somnolent Samantha, the character that Jon Westling, president of Boston University, invented in 1995. (Thanks to Zosha Stuckey and Lois Agnew, who examine this case more closely in an essay in the journal *Open Words*). Westling's story was about a student named Samantha, who had a documented learning disability. In Westling's story, Samantha is a caricature who greedily demands extra time on assignments and exams, copies of notes from lectures, a seat at the front of the class, and a separate room in which to take tests; most memorably, she also warns him that she will fall asleep in his class, and thus will need someone to take notes while she is asleep—thus he calls her "somnolent" Samantha. Later, Westling admitted that the story was a lie. But he argued that Somnolent Samantha characterized the unreasonable expectations universities were being held to by opportunistic students and the unfair challenges administrators and teachers faced in responding to their mandate to accommodate disability. His argument was, basically, that these students were milking the system and probably didn't belong in university at all if they couldn't play by the "normal" rules. Somnolent Samantha and other fictional students like her are key characters invented through discourse about disability in higher education. These students are the "real" problem, Westling argued, despite the fact that he had just invented one.

Samantha is much like the "Johnny" of Myra Linden and Arthur Whimbey's 1990 *Why Johnny Can't Write*, an unfortunate classic in writing scholarship, a book that begins with the warning that "Johnny's Country Is Losing Business," and goes on to strongly advocate for a series of sentence-combining and text-reconstruction exercises to fix Johnny and the economy. But imaginary college and university students are more common than you'd think. They pop up everywhere.

This book would be incomplete without both a deeper investigation of the students who get invented through the backlash to accommodations in higher education, and a deeper investigation of the invention of the ideal students who stand in their inverse image. So I'll introduce two more characters, each reinvented and reshaped in unique ways by recent attention to multimodality and multiliteracies. To keep things simple, I'll make everyone a Samantha of some sort.

Super Samantha

The first character might be named Super Samantha. This student appears in some form in almost all of the literature about multimodality, and quite a bit of the scholarship about the use of technology in the classroom. Super Samantha is much better at nonprint literacies than all of her peers and most of her teachers. She is technologically savvy, crafty, and has mastered modes that her elders haven't even heard of (yet). She is Mark Zuckerberg and Doogie Howser and Dora the Explorer with a brand-new backpack.

Samantha, very notably, is a spectacle. As Rachel Riedner writes of such spectacular stories, "like melodramas, spectacles are written to obscure more complex and nuanced stories. The shock they elicit displaces complex situations, shaping our response through astonishment and surprise rather than through sustained attention. . . . no effort is called for to shift how we respond" (105). Somnolent and Super Samantha are spectacles of neoliberalism, in Riedner's scheme: they are in fact the only two types of student neoliberalism needs. One is totally flexible to a wide range of uses and values within capitalism. One is a total drain on the system and thus disposable.

Bronwyn Williams writes obliquely about this super student in his introduction to Cindy Selfe's edited collection *Multimodal Composition*, suggesting that he sometimes finds this student's "energy and creativity unnerving" (xi). In short, this student is Super, because they already have multimodal literacies that far outstrip those of their teachers; thus, they are also Scary because these teachers aren't sure how to teach them. In either case, they hide more nuanced stories and more realistic roles for students.

Selfe has looked extensively at how technological literacy has been characterized in the media, government, and in our scholarship. She would likely say that Super Samantha belongs in the overdone discourse or "story" of what she might call multimodality as a literacy boon: "in the hands of [Super Samantha, multimodality] can help us make the world a better place." In this way, Super Samantha is not scary in the horror-film way—she is scary in a way that should be celebrated. Selfe would likely say that Super Samantha is linked to "science, economic prosperity, education, capitalism, and democracy," and thus her story "has a potent cumulative power" (Technology and Literacy, 27). But, again, she is an idealized character, and she is invoked most often to show that universities do not have the educational resources, infrastructure, or pedagogical skill to accommodate her in the classroom.

Regardless, Super Samantha is in the driver's seat when it comes to designing multimodal pedagogy. As Gunther Kress writes, multimodality is born of the idea that "we do not yet have a theory which allows us to understand and account for the world of communication as it is now" (Multimodality, 7). This world will belong to Super Samantha. The ideal that she presents propels us to create learning opportunities that live up to her potential: build it because she is already here. For instance, Stuart Selber, in *Multiliteracies for a Digital Age*, uses "a portrait of the ideal multiliterate student" to lay out his argument for educational change (22).[2]

In some stories, she is all of our students already. Selfe, in an article coauthored with Gail Hawisher and others, profiles a student named Brittney who "authored web sites as a child," and saw computers being as essential as air (Hawisher et. al. 656). Brittney's story shows "how little teachers of English, composition and communication know about the many literacies students bring to the classroom" (Hawisher et. al.676). This student, then, is not molded by education, but rather bursts through the doors of the classroom and demands its reshaping.[3] The literature is full of further case studies, and example work, from multimodally advanced students (students with advanced multiliteracy).

Super Samantha's multimodality, however, is strikingly visual. Perhaps we shouldn't be surprised. We do live in an "ocularcentric" culture—that is, one in which visual images dominate (Jay, 344). But there is a distinct lack of exploration of, for instance, tactile modes of creation in the classroom. This omission might tie into what Evan Watkins suggests is the dominance of visual culture in an "attention economy" in which teachers become resource managers who need to train students to create a "product" that gains value only if people will pay attention to it (94). Creating a truly diverse range of modes, or creating a redundant array of modes, doesn't have the same value.

Especially in a time of economic crisis, in the panic of postindustrialism, as manufacturing jobs disappear and new "knowledge jobs" (or "attention jobs") need to be created, Super Samantha is a powerful character. She is never invoked uncritically—but she seems to be always invoked. Super Samantha can be considered a product or even a flag-bearer of fast capitalism, a logic stressing the need for constant change, flexibility, and adaptation, particularly in modes of expression. Fast capitalism is also a logic that uses this rhetoric to encourage compliance and to sort workers.[4] Simply, when capitalism demands speed and flexibility, it is mostly in service of more efficiently exploiting workers. So while a postindustrial society (and a post-Fordist one, where the rigidity and uniformity of manufacturing is less prevalent) might or maybe should help us to de-emphasize things like the strict time regimes of academia, there are always other demands to be made.

In other stories, Super Samantha lives in India or China, where a new generation of savvy students is mastering all of the skills that North American students are not, and leaving these domestic students behind. She is then marked also as being governed by different political, religious, or social rules, each of which somehow frees her to develop her superiority in ways that North American students cannot. As Kress warns, "a new theory of text is essential to meet the demands of culturally plural societies in a globalizing world" ("Genres," 186). Meanwhile, in North America, the question of whether multiliteracies would accommodate multilingualism continues to hinge on economic and cultural values that recognize foreign language usage as either only a skill, or as a threat to national sovereignty: "skill versus sedition" (Lo Bianco, n.p.). Multiliteracy gets framed as something North American students need to acquire in the name of nationalism and economic competition. North America needs to globalize and become more culturally plural—again only, somewhat ironically, in the name of nationalism and economic competition. So we witness a sort of literacy protectionism—the shielding of domestic assets from foreign competition by taxing imports; the shielding of domestic student abilities from foreign competition by taxing the import of multiliteracy, especially when language difference is part of the equation.

Super Samantha is also a character that many in the disability rights community know well, even if at first we don't recognize her. It is the specter of just such a student that leads to a backlash against accessible education and things like the ADA: if you accommodate all students and treat the classroom with a democratic and egalitarian ethic, then you could be holding back our Super students. That's un-American!

It's un-Canadian too, it seems. An administrator at my own university visited a department meeting recently to give a "state of the university address" to myself and my colleagues. The thought that the administrator left us with was this: Is it time for special classes for our best students? What this individual meant, in my opinion, was that we needed not just honors plans or specializations that only a few students could get into, and not even just the usual selectivity of admissions. What they meant was: Do we need to create distinct tiers within the university wherein the smartest students could be kept away from the riffraff? My university, Waterloo, is a Canadian (and world) leader in engineering, math, and computer science. The administrator, then, was distilling an emerging institutional ethic: we need to let a lot of students in because we need the money; but then we'll also need ways to ensure that these new individuals don't impede the progress of all of our Super Samanthas. Again, any teacher could likely look around their own campus and find similar programs, programs that could be similarly questioned: Are these programs about bringing the brightest together, or about keeping them away from the least bright? It is clear that one group will be tolerated for their tuition; but the university's real priorities are built around the other.

In the disability community, there is awareness that accommodations for students with disabilities have traditionally been cast as happening at the cost of all other students, and particularly at the cost of Super students. A *New York Times* article suggested, for instance, that such accommodations have "subverted the goal of education" and have "discouraged students from discovering their strengths, and instead encouraged them to get ahead based on their weaknesses" (Sternberg, A23). Super Samantha fools even the best teachers into believing that the entire education system must be oriented around her. This orientation should then cue educators into the realization that modes and literacies come from bodies. (Remember: If rhetoric is the circulation of discourse through the body, then spaces and institutions cannot be disconnected from the bodies within them, the bodies they selectively exclude, and the bodies that actively intervene to reshape them.)

As Charles Murray has shown, North American colleges and universities have been tremendously successful at sorting citizens, with the top 10 U.S. schools sucking up 20 percent of the top group of students—based on standardized tests. This sorting then also leads to what he calls "cognitive homogamy: when individuals with similar cognitive ability have children," as discussed previously (61). Then this allows Murray to map every zip code in the United States based on education and income and recognize a small number of "SuperZips" to show that "the college sorting machine replicates itself with remarkable fidelity as the residential sorting machine" (88). The connection between Super students and something like SuperZips, however, is rarely made by teachers or administrators. As Evan Watkins argues, "one of the more dangerous assumptions" of the expansion of "adjectival literacies" (his term for the multiplication of different types of literacy, most often linked to "professional" opportunities and prestige) "with their maximizing of student/teacher educational freedoms" is that they transform "a particular institution into one of the prestigious stars that visibly succeed" or for students to likewise become "stars" (Literacy, 159). The evolving neoliberal economy needs a few prestigious schools to provide "just-in-time" flexible labor and "human capital" but it is also "structured to lose excess people—both students and workers" (Literacy, 158).

So Super Samantha also possesses a kind of magical invisibility cloak. When she appears, she is able to sweep important considerations about socioeconomic class, race, gender, and linguistic difference away. When Super Samantha is invoked, and the demand is made that instructors adapt curriculum to catch up to her, we can also conveniently ignore the fact that access to the technologies and means that facilitate multimodality is not distributed equally. For every SuperZip with a direct line to the Ivy League, there are other Zips with pipelines to prison. So long as we are straining to change for the ideal student, and for a new knowledge economy, we can ignore the inequities that may have positioned her ahead of the pack to begin with. We can ignore the economic realities that make Super students temporarily valuable. And we can definitely avoid wasting time on the stragglers.[5]

Slow Samantha

This brings us to the second character: Slow Samantha. She is the sister or cousin to Super Samantha. Unlike Super Samantha, who is most often seen as an independent and self-determined individual, Slow Samantha is a composite, invoked to represent an entire group or population of students, and to represent troubling trends that multimodal pedagogy might sweep in to heroically alleviate. In the end, Slow Samantha is a threat. As one *Time* magazine article put it, "the rising numbers of learning-disabled students have altered classroom dynamics in ways that harm average kids' ability to learn" at the K-12 level (Ratner, n.p.). Further, the article suggests that these learning disabled students cost nine billion dollars a year to educate. The suggestion is that this is badly wasted money. This calculation is a kind of eugenic economics, because no one ever talks about the billions spent on other groups of students as anything like a waste.[6] Jasbir Puar asks: "Which debilitated bodies can be reinvigorated for neoliberalism, and which cannot?" (153). More simply, the United States likely spends over eight hundred billion dollars a year on education (or 4.8% of its GDP).[7] That makes nine billion actually seem quite small. And then one has to ask: why single this group of students out as a cost rather than as an investment?

What we have seen over the past 150 years of disability history is that, during periods of economic collapse or downturn, people with disabilities are the first to be constructed as drains or threats—Susan Schweik's work on *Ugly Laws*, or David Serlin's history of postwar prosthetics, shows how industrial capitalism picked up or put down disabled bodies according to its needs. The ways in which disability is socially constructed in contemporary society can also be seen as, from top-to-bottom, economic. Disability is an object of charity rather than part of the social contract, the disabled body must be made productive or expendable, exhibited or warehoused for profit, the disability itself must be easily monetized—all of these things ensure that disability can be easily controlled in order to absorb or expel citizens from status positions.[8] The work of Chris Chapman, Liat Ben Moshe, and Allison Carey on disability and incarceration powerfully shows one such way this economic expendability works from below.[9] The university is another perfect example of such an economic ordering of disability "from above." That is, more simply, incarceration warehouses and disciplines certain groups disproportionately, and uses disability and disablement as part of this work. Colleges and universities support this work, but they also work to suspend opportunities for disabled people, or use forms of disablement to suspend opportunities and privileges for marginalized groups.

More simply, which type of body will our current academic economy choose to take advantage of next, and which type of body will be cast aside? On college campuses, an individual learning disability makes you a drain; but a collective lack of multiliteracy calls for an investment. In turn, administrators, teachers, and commentators will take the liberty to question or ridicule "new" disabilities claimed by students. But they will also invent disabled students as straw-figures and scapegoats.

Slow Samantha is the direct descendent of Johnny-Can't-Read and Johnny-Can't-Write. In fact, a *New Republic* article on this topic actually remixed this classic title: "Why Johnny Can't Read, Write or Sit Still." In the article, Ruth Shalit argues that disability accommodations in higher education have created a "new frontier, the learning disability as an opportunistic tautology" (244). In this invented scheme, we aren't looking at multimodality, but instead we are looking at a strong back-lash against an expanding range of disabilities. Multi-disability. As Shalit writes, "as the ranks of the learning-disabled swell, so too do the number of boutique diagnoses" (244). She goes on to incredulously list dyscal-culia, dysgraphia, Attention Deficit Disorder (ADD), Attention Deficit Hyperactivity Disorder (ADHD), Oppositional Defiant Disorder (ODD), dysphasia, dyssemia, and dysrationalia before she concludes that "these neo-disabilities are likely to strike the nonspecialist as an exercise in pathologizing [regular] childhood [and youth] behavior, and the non-specialist would be on to something" (244). Robert Worth, writing in the *Washington Monthly*, sees this as a class conspiracy: he argues that we have "inflated the meaning of 'disability,' encouraging wealthier families to capitalize on their [children's] weaknesses at the expense of their peers" (n.p.). He wishes, instead, that disability policy could be "merely a mat-ter of accommodating physically disabled kids" and thus return to being "a relatively straightforward affair" (n.p.).

While we are urged to race to accommodate the multiple literacies that Super Samantha introduces to the classroom, we are urged to dis-miss and derogate the needs of Slow Samantha. Slow Samantha may not be as powerful a character as Super Samantha in our scholarship about multimodality, but she is present persistently. Hawisher and Selfe begin an acceptance speech with this warning: "Today, if students cannot write to the screen . . . they may be incapable of functioning effectively as liter-ate citizens in a growing number of social spheres" (642). Their warning is later carefully qualified. But others are less cautious, more willing to invoke an epidemic of multi-illiteracy. There is urgency to this epidemic: Robert Davis and Mark Shadle argue that we need to "prepare students to compose flexibly in a world that will present them with discursive occasions, genres, and technologies that cannot be seen but will break upon them in an instant, like a rogue wave upon a surfer" (3). And there are diagnoses in this epidemic. Frank Zingrone perhaps distills this most simply: "a one-medium user is the new illiterate" (237).[10] Slow Samantha is a kind of human vacuum, and whenever she appears in rhetoric about multimodality, she is defined by what she can't do—and what she can't do stands in for deficits of the entire educational and social system.[11]

In this way, the rhetoric is normative, with the norm defined as "a polemical concept which negatively qualifies: the abnormal, while logically second, is existentially first" (Canguilhem, 243). To norm is to employ a logic of negation. Roland Barthes, John Fiske, and Patricia Williams have all written about this process of "exnomination" as it applies to race. As Jeffrey Melnick and Rachel Rubin argue, "the practice of racial naming" always entails "the unnaming of whiteness itself as a racial identity" (265). Siobhan Somerville argues that "culture anchors whiteness in the visible epistemology of black skin" (21). This contrast is also how normativity works: an elaborate taxonomy of abnormality is created and applied. Ability is anchored and erected through the labeling of disability. Others have written about how such a logic exists with the literacy/illiteracy binary: we track illiteracy rates; literacy is existentially second to illiteracy (access Connie Kendall). Mental health is also an exnomination of mental illness or mental disability. We act as though what we are talking about is health, and this conversation will be generative, but really it is health that is being demanded. The New London Group coined the term multiliteracy as part of an argument for multimodality. But that argument is based on a lack, on the absence of enough of this learning and of these learners. Slow Struggling Samantha reveals how multi-illiteracy precedes any concept of multiliteracy.

What we get is an intersection of a sort of rhetorical "literacy craft" and "ability craft"—ways of insinuating that a lack of literacy or a lack of modality are actually deficits, biological deficits, and that if you don't have these things, you are disabled.[12] As Elspeth Stuckey wrote, "The face of illiteracy is less and less linguistic" (101). That is, illiteracy is now directly affiliated with immigrants, with young mothers, with inmates, with indigenous peoples, with the jobless, with those on welfare, and so on. Thus illiteracy gathers power from what it can be associated with, and it also crucially gathers definition from these affiliations; it is magnetically affiliative. Other downward comparisons stick to illiteracy. A lack of literacy, like a lack of "modality," can thus be a way to insinuate a biological lack or difference, a disability, without coming out and saying it, or writing it.

Slow Samantha is at all times defined by incapacities, inabilities, and lack of function. This concept of slowed literacy also has a eugenic history. As Christina Cogdell shows us, the creation of streamlined fonts and the inclusion of photographs in magazines such as *Time* created speed and an "efficiency . . . produced through the processes of 'natural selection' that had weeded out all that was too 'slow' and 'cumbersome' and increased the tempo at which a text could be read" (145). This increased efficiency led to the idea of "greater rapidity and intelligence brought about by evolution" based on the idea that "certain linguistic developments evidenced racial superiority" (Cogdell, 144). A culture that could read quickly, and multimodally access information on the page, could advance. To be slow was to be illiterate, and to be illiterate was to be (cognitively and evolutionarily) slow. Both concepts work together within larger eugenic frameworks in which the speed of thought is aligned with racial and biological progress.[13] If we aren't maxing out all the different ways our brains might be engaged, then our brains are somehow deficient (individually and across the population).

The call for multimodal pedagogies rises out of warnings about increasing multi-illiteracies, and thus Slow Samantha's incapabilities seem to multiply: there are seemingly no limits to the number of social spheres for which our students will be unprepared and from which they will be exempted if they don't max out all of their literacies by maxing out all of the possible, interconnected modes of expression. The New London Group talks about the "social futures" that multimodality might make possible: but these have a tone of warning wrapped around their optimism. Even after the concept of multimodality opens up an expanded realm of literate possibilities, the very idea of multimodality remains based on the idea that we have nations of Slow Samanthas. The social future she is prepared for is not very bright at all.

Hawisher and Selfe, in the above-mentioned essay and in other work, are strongly focused on the social consequences of literacy debates—and thus the consequences of modality debates, too. So the very basis for the focus on multimodality includes a blanket awareness that the focus on traditional print literacies privileges one group and one avenue to learning. There is a theoretical way to look at this: the New London Group argues that all learning happens multimodally—as Gunther Kress writes, our senses' interaction "guarantees the multimodality of our semiotic world." Yet, "the selection and concentration by a culture on one or several modes (and the non-selection of others) opens up and facilitates [our] bodily engagement with the world in specific ways" while closing down others (111). There is also a practical way to look at this: in the classroom, we have focused on very few literacies and modes for expression for far too long. It follows that students who think and communicate differently have been suppressed and silenced through our teaching.

But immediately following this argument, however it is posed, we almost always get the connected argument that because of this enduring mono-literacy, we are left with classrooms full of Slow students—but now, instead of the old illiteracy, we have a new range of multi-illiteracies. What remains, recognizable to those in disability studies, is the creation of a stigma that can be applied to students based on a perceived deficit.

Importantly, Slow Samantha is also the product of a much larger educational paradigm—one that demands that all skills be quantifiable and testable. This demand means that the multimodal student must max out all literacies and modes as much as possible, all of the time. Modality is not about choice. But if it isn't about choice, then it isn't about access. Further, we know that teachers generally "miss opportunities to incorporate non-Eurocentric scholarship to normalize the 'what' of multimodal composition" (access Yumani Davis). So the only multiliteracies that come to matter are those already dominant, already sanctioned, and already filtered through English.

In the "good old days," something like "cultural literacy," made famous by E. D. Hirsch's arguments about—and lists of—the essential cultural facts every citizen should know, could sort society. You either knew the names of Shakespeare's plays or you did not. But now that access to this sort of cultural information is just a click away, it becomes more difficult to classify society based on access to information. The push for multiliteracies, then, shifts the framework. Now there is an increasing list of modes (most often technological but also increasingly artisanal) that one must master. This listing, in and of itself, is relatively unproblematic. It is good to have access to these varied ways of learning. But multimodality and multiliteracies pedagogy has more often emphasized panic about multiple illiteracies, demanded that students learn to max out all literacies, engaged with new modes and mediums and genres without interrogating their accessibility, and failed to foreground students' agentive role in forming and transforming avenues for expression.

The problem, for example, with much of the rhetoric of the New London Group is the implicit argument that, as mentioned earlier, in each individual learner, the more modes engaged, the better—and this is rooted in much of the underexamined cognitivist emphasis of the group's work.[14] I would argue that we do not all have the same proclivity, desire, or ability to develop all of our sensory engagements—nor do the forms of sensory engagement necessarily align with single senses.

We should encourage the multiple engagement of senses and learning pathways, but we should not map them and add them up toward a multimodal IQ. There is a difference between engaging multiple modes and offering students choices of modes.[15]

Critical Multimodality

Joddy Murray states that multimodality "is a compositional form . . . which, coincidentally, happens to be closer to the way humans think" than discursive text is (185). This closeness may be somewhat truthful—but this does not mean that multimodality will allow for expression uncomplicated by unequal and unpredictable affordances, proclivities and abilities. In short, multimodality should not make us forget everything that either poststructuralism or the disability rights movement has taught us.

To begin with, amid all of the panic and excitement around multimodality, very few teachers have paid any attention at all to the ways that these new modes multiply possibilities for inaccessibility. Instead, they create what Stephanie Kerschbaum calls multimodal inhospitality: "many multimodal texts are not commensurable across modes, [and] inaccessible multimodal spaces are too often remedied by a problematic turn to the retrofit [and] texts and environments are rarely flexible enough to be manipulated by users" (in Oswal et al., n.p.). Thus "multimodal inhospitality occurs when the design and production of multimodal texts and environments persistently ignore access except as a retrofit" (in Oswal et al., n.p.). Janine Butler adds that "to increase the potential for making multimodal compositions inclusive, we need to synchronize modes so that different bodies and senses can access meaning" (n.p.). In my own field of composition, we have acknowledged that composition (as a process) has become increasingly multimodal (Yancey; Ball). This acknowledgment means that the tools and avenues of composing need to be reconsidered in terms of accessibility. Which bodies can compose which texts, under what circumstances? But we also need to realize that, even when a composition is primarily text based, its reception is bound to be multimodal—it will be accessed through screen-readers, enlarged, read across platforms, translated, and so on. Moreover, in what ways will the text move, move through, or move past (which) bodies? Reception needs to be reconsidered in terms of accessibility—this expands the author's responsibility. But the means of distribution and reproduction also need to be reconsidered in terms of accessibility. Which bodies can take up texts and move (with) them? If we understand rhetoric as the circulation of power and discourse through the body, then we'd want to view this through a wide range of possible bodies, or even the widest range of possible bodies.

So a starting point for any multiliteracy or multimodality pedagogy is, as with any other form of teaching, a questioning of access.

In my discipline of composition and rhetoric, the landmark Conference on College Composition and Communication's "Student's Right to Their Own Language" argued that varieties of language use do not derive from "supposed differences in intelligence or physiology" and that the "variety of dialects enriches the language" (Scott et al., 717). We must extend this argument to recognize that engagements with different modes of meaning-making does not map onto differences of intelligence or physiology either. Students must have the right to their own literacies, learning styles, and modes of expression—literacies, styles, and modes that it is the job of the academy to recognize, validate, and make space for, therefore enriching our cultures, ourselves, our classrooms, and our disciplines.

Just like Somnolent Samantha, my Samanthas are fictitious. However, recognizing the ways that these characters are created in service of particular cultural narratives is important—especially as they impact the roles that we make available to any student. Multimodal pedagogies might move forward by recognizing that an expanded range of expressive possibilities, instead of creating new ways to be inferior, and instead of hiding inequities under the costume of progress, offer new contact points for engaging with the difficult work of teaching and learning.

Putting together this chapter with the last chapter on retrofits, we can understand that so many academic accommodations are shifts or even redundancies in modes: copies of lecture notes, a transcript for a video, the ability to be tested orally instead of in writing, and so on. But why, when one group asks to shift modes, or for information to be given across more than one mode, are they deficient, asking for something special? Why, then, when another group shifts or repeats modes, are they constructed as Super? In the next chapter, I will explore the ways that we might better teach all students if and when these redundancies, shifts, and multiplications in modes of engagement become part of the Universal Design of teaching.

CHAPTER FOUR

Universal Design

———— ❦ ————

Margaret Price, from her book *Mad at School*, about mental disability and higher education:

"Rhetoric is not simply the words we speak or write or sign, nor is it simply what we look like or sound like. It is who we are, and beyond that, it is who we are allowed to be." (27)

So this brings us to our third metaphor: Universal Design (UD). In explaining Universal Design I want to emphasize the importance of the priority and activity of Universal Design as a process and mode of becoming. As Ronald Mace, one of the founders of the concept, wrote, "universal design is the design of products and environments to be usable by all people, to the greatest extent possible, without the need for adaptation or specialized design" (1).[1] UD has gone through what linguists call a "nominalization." That is, it has been changed from a verb into a noun—a solid, clearly defined thing, rather than a process. But in this chapter, I will try to reanimate UD as a verb.

The UD movement was first an architectural movement that worked against the exclusion of people with disabilities, and argued that instead of temporarily accommodating difference, physical structures should be designed with a wide range of citizens in mind, planning for the active involvement of all. Every year, awards are given for the most Universally Designed buildings, and specific features such as level entrances and layouts, motion-detecting lights, nonslip surfaces, lever-style handles instead of doorknobs are all Universally Designed features. UD then also has become a major force in the design of smaller products and applications like, famously, OXO Good Grip kitchen utensils—originally designed to be used regardless of strength and dexterity. The result has been "the creation of an internationally recognised brand [and] 100 design awards. As for profits, in 1991, two years after product development began, the [OXO] company made $3 million in sales. Since then sales have increased by 50 percent each year" (Center for Excellence in Universal Design).

Principles for Universal Design, developed by a team of researchers at North Carolina State University, and now widely accepted as (at least somewhat) definitive of the concept, include:

> Equitable Use: The design is useful and marketable to people with diverse abilities.
>
> Flexibility in Use: The design accommodates a wide range of individual preferences and abilities.
>
> Simple and Intuitive Use: Use of the design is easy to understand, regardless of the user's experience, knowledge, language skills, or current concentration level.
>
> Perceptible Information: The design communicates necessary information effectively to the user, regardless of ambient conditions or the user's sensory abilities.
>
> Tolerance for Error: The design minimizes hazards and the adverse consequences of accidental or unintended actions.
>
> Low Physical Effort: The design can be used efficiently and comfortably and with a minimum of fatigue.
>
> Size and Space for Approach and Use: Appropriate size and space is provided for approach, reach, manipulation, and use regardless of user's body size, posture, or mobility. (Center for Universal Design)[2]

I want to point out that Universal Design, as a list, and as applied solely to the physical environment, as in this example, looks a lot like a set of specifications. Indeed, UD is often interpreted in this way. Yet UD, registered as action, is a way to move. In some ways, it is also a worldview. Universal Design is not a tailoring of the environment to marginal groups; it is a form of hope, a manner of trying.

Universal Design is a means of thinking through multiple sites, while also acknowledging that fixed locations, like the steep steps in the "approach" to Rensselaer Polytechnic Institute discussed at the beginning of this book, fade, fall, and disintegrate, even as new passive-aggressive ramps and curb cuts to nowhere are built. The push toward the universal is a push toward seeing space as open to multiple possibilities, as being in process. More simply, the universal is an acknowledgment that our design practices have long been biased. Take for example the fact that many people find the buildings in which they work too hot or too cold. Why does this happen? Because building climates were designed based on the body of a 154 pound male (Kingma and van Marken Lichtenbelt). The temperature is just one very small example of design bias—bias in which a normate body was the end goal and end user for almost all design.[3] To be more universal, we need to design for a much more diverse group of people.

As mentioned in the beginning of the book, to a certain degree all disabilities on college campuses are invisible—until an accommodation is granted, they have no legal reality. But so-called invisible disabilities are particularly fraught in an educational setting in which students with disabilities are already routinely and systematically constructed as faking it, jumping a queue, or asking for an advantage. The stigma of disability is something that drifts all over—it can be used to insinuate inferiority, revoke privilege, and step society very freely. But the rights that come with disability do not drift very easily at all. Ableism drifts—so must accommodations and access. When we recognize physical inaccessibility we can and should read intellectual and social inaccessibility into this space. We currently live in a society in which one single disability can be linked to any other disability in a negative way. But could we live in a society in which the accessibility we create for one person can also lead us to broaden and expand accessibility for all? On the way to this world, we at least have to recognize that physical access is not "enough"—it is not where accessibility should stop.

Universal Design responds to the idea, here expressed by Lennard Davis, that "what is universal in life, if there are universals, is the experience of the limitations of the body" (Bending, 32). Difference, Davis asserts, "is what we all have in common" (Bending, 26). This is not to say that we are all disabled, but to show that "we are all non-standard," disabled by oppression and injustice (Bending, 32). In response to this, we can either disavow our difference and project it upon others, or we can join in an "ethic of liberation" (Bending, 29). Davis suggests that disability epistemology, or "dismodernism," to borrow his phrase, shows us that identity is not fixed but malleable, that technology is not separate but part of the body, that dependence, not individual independence, is the rule (Bending, 26). Further, through UD, in the words of Rosemarie Garland-Thomson, "disability can be a narrative resource that does not trade the present in on the future" and instead "contributes a narrative of a genuinely open future, one not controlled by the objectives, expectations, and understandings of the present. Perhaps counterintuitively, rather than dictating a diminished future, disability opens a truly unpredictable, even unimaginable, one" ("Case For," 352). Design for disability and benefit all.

As Sean Zdenek writes about the growing acceptance of captioning as a facet of the Universal Design of media, when it "enters the mainstream . . . [it] becomes more natural and less strange, more universal and less marginal, more central to our theories, pedagogies and . . . habits and less likely to be overlooked or forgotten" (301). The same can be said about many other aspects of Universal Design: they are means of reorienting not just priorities but also conversations and theories. I like Universal Design mainly because of the verb—design. This active dimension suggests that UD is a way to plan, to foresee, to imagine the future. The "Universal" of UD also suggests that disability is something that is always a part of our worldview. Thus, when UD is successful, it is hopeful and realistic—allowing teachers to structure space and pedagogy in the broadest possible manner. Universal Design is not about buildings, it is about building—building community, building better pedagogy, building opportunities for agency. It is a way to move.

Deep, Transformative, Tolerant, Redundant

I should clarify that, in the historical transition between UD as an architectural concept to UD as a concept for the design of classrooms, or even social spaces, there was also a transition away from simply seeing disability as being about wheelchair access. Star Ford, in addressing the fact that almost all discourse about access and UD defaults to thinking about physical disability, developed the concept of "deep accessibility," creating "five levels of accessibility, extending the familiar notion of wheelchair access to the sensory and cognitive levels of accessibility" (n.p.). I will summarize these five levels here:

1. Movement—getting there—how we get to an event or class.
2. Sense—being there—how we access the material, the conversation.

3. Architecture—orienting—how the space and layout structure our belonging and understanding.

4. Communication—how we join the conversation, engage, understand and are understood, what Zahari Richter calls "communicative access" ("Some Notes," n.p.).

5. Agency—autonomy—how we can come to have a shaping role in the event or class, as well as the right to define our own identity and involvement.

In this scheme we move from the idea that access is only about getting there and getting in—to a library, a classroom, a conference, a protest—to the fact that once we are there, we need to be able to perceive all that is going on, sort important information from noise, and sense the action without delay or undue stress. Then, we also need to have ways for all bodies and minds to understand the orientation of the architecture—to understand its ideologies and affordances as well as how it might divert bodies and minds, to understand what the buildings mean. And we all need to be able to communicate. Then, finally, we all need to be able to ask our questions, make our ideas known, and share in discourse in a shaping way.

For UD to work we need to have all five levels of access, all the way up to the level of agency and autonomy, the idea that all users should shape the space. This interdependence links to what Elizabeth Brewer, Melanie Yergeau, and Cynthia Selfe call "transformative access." They suggest that "there is a profound difference between consumptive access and transformative access. The former allows people to enter a space or access a text. The latter questions and re-thinks the very construct of allowing" (153–54). Transformative access, then, sees space, social space, and learning space, as being in process—and sees all as involved in designing that space.

If we were to look at some of the foundational principles of UD and apply them beyond the physical sphere, we could begin to understand how deep accessibility and transformative access would work in a classroom. For instance, let's examine the concept of tolerance for error, meaning that "the design minimizes hazards and the adverse consequences of accidental or unintended actions" (Center for Universal Design). We could and should understand something like the "auto correct" function on a phone as an example of this tolerance for error.[4] A more physical example is a lever door handle that can be moved upward, downward, pushed or pulled to open a door; a door that swings in both directions, and that has an access button for a powered opening (and that access button is large, easy to find, and easy to push). In this way, tolerance for error overlaps with the UD concept of redundancy: if there are fewer ways to be wrong or to make mistakes, then there also become many ways to be right. So, if the goal is to understand and to show how well you understand a difficult concept in class, there should be multiple avenues to get to that understanding and to convey it. There should be multiple ways to open that door even if they are redundant.[5]

Let me further explore what the door handle or the auto-correct metaphor can do for social interaction or for the classroom. In my own classroom, where there is often a reliance on discussion, I create "tolerance for error" by making sure that students who don't want to raise their hands and respond in the moment can have time to write questions and comments down (on note cards) and submit them to be read aloud anonymously. That removes some of the difficulty of trying out a new idea on the spot in an intense social situation—where the fear often is that they will get something wrong. It creates time for students to think through their ideas and answers and use writing (or an alternative modality) to compose them. More time can be created by asking for the cards to be completed between classes rather than during them. Instead of using discussion as an informal and camouflaged form of testing, what I end up getting is more and better input from students. This is what I wanted, to begin with. I break down the idea that the only thinking students can do is in the few moments in which the teacher waits for them to respond, or even in the 50–80 minutes of a class session. They can do more and better thinking if given more time and different ways to contribute. Isn't that what we want (at least most of the time): more and better thinking?[6]

This strategy also creates "equitable use" in that it recognizes diverse abilities. There are redundant or repetitive or duplicated ways to take part, but no one way is privileged over the others. The raise-your-hand modality isn't the best way to allow all students to show what they know and to shape what we can all know together. There is also "flexibility in use" in that there can still be the old form of discussion in addition to this new mode. There is a "lower physical effort" in that there is more space created for quiet, more time given for students to process and compose their thoughts, and less emphasis on exchanges that can be anxiety producing for some students. While I may not be creating "size and space for approach and use," I am creating an important analogue:

more time for students to approach the discussion and the ideas, more time to use them in their own ways.

This note-card technique can also be used during public talks or lectures and conference presentations—places where putting your hand up to ask a question can be even more difficult. In this case, many of the same benefits can be realized—benefits to deep accessibility, and benefits that involve more people in transforming what is being learned within the larger group, rather than simply creating ramps for people to access the content but not reshape it.

On Futurity

The example above disrupts a relatively extreme bias of academia: the idea that learning has to happen in scheduled bursts and limited openings. But it also disrupts the idea that knowledge, in the classroom, is located in the teacher. This idealization of the teacher, as well as the mechanization of learning, are legacies that UD can seek to challenge.

Yet as theorists such as Christina Cogdell have shown, for much of the 20th century, the focus of design has been on streamlining, on speed, and on normative ideal types—ideal bodies for which designers sought not only to create products for but sought to sell products to create. That is, design itself was an extension of eugenics—in the middle part of the 20th century, "designers' rhetoric strongly suggests that their conceptions of 'ideal types' in product design were intricately, ideologically entwined with eugenicists' pursuits of the same goal in social and biological design" (Cogdell, 213). This idealization is basically the opposite of the design of products for the broadest range of users and uses. A factory, a vacuum, a car were all designed with an "ideal human" in mind and as their goal (Cogdell, 213). More simply, you didn't make something just to be of use to a consumer. You made things that in part *formed* ideal consumers. The university was also designed, architecturally, with the ideal human in mind and as its goal. This conditions the spaces and the times of education.[7]

On the college or university campus, we know that the steps are steep, and they are also steeped in tradition. Many universities make the argument that steep steps are stylistically desirable, that they fit with the template, the architectural fingerprint of the school. These arguments show the ways that in the construction and maintenance of the steep steps there is also a latent argument about aesthetics (access Hunter, "Out of Sight, Out of Mind: Disability and the Aesthetics of Landscape Architecture"). Change, then, is framed as a deformation, and a transgression of not only space but time. The Rensselaer approach that we began the book with, built of marble and in a Greek style, was not really a new construction in any way. (The crumbling of these steps, over time, reveals the tenuousness of any boundary—it also shows us that as boundaries fall, they can be replaced by an even more insurmountable landscape.) As I mentioned earlier, other campuses, many of them built around churches, similarly rely on steps not just as architectural details, but as symbolic social centerpieces of university life —traditional university life.

The point is that students with disabilities are excluded not just from campus space, but from the entirety of collegiate history and lore. The retrofit is, as I said, an after-the-fact construction. It is always supplemental—always not-original. The retrofit is additional. But as a supplement, to retrofit is to fix in some way. Like eugenic design, a retrofit can be meant not to fit a need, but to make its user perform and behave in a particular way, often in a constrained way. Unfortunately, this fixing provides little opportunity for continued refitting, for process. Yet Universal Design is a philosophy that, I hope to show, can provide a heuristic framework that makes disability essential to embodiment—it is a way of looking toward an inclusive future.

David Mitchell and Sharon Snyder argue that UD "organizes a disability time and place by shifting educational environments according to the demands of its peculiar, nonnormative logistics" and this "promises to widen the arena of embodiment for all" (Biopolitics, 93).

While the "universal" of UD is problematic (access discussion below), I believe that within the concept of Universal Design we should focus on the verb—design. In this way, and in the spirit of Mitchell and Snyder's "disability time and place" UD becomes a way to plan, to foresee, to imagine the future (Biopolitics, 93).

As Alison Kafer writes: "how one understands disability in the present determines how one imagines disability in the future" (2). But she clarifies that disability has a vexed futurity:

The value of a future that includes disabled people goes unrecognized, while the value of a disability-free future is seen as self-evident;

and second, the political nature of disability, namely its position as a category to be contested and debated, goes unacknowledged. The second failure of recognition makes possible the first; casting disability as monolithic fact of the body, as beyond the realm of the political and therefore beyond the realm of debate or dissent, makes it impossible to imagine disability and disability futures differently. (3)

We must connect Kafer's argument back to eugenics and the reshaping of how North Americans thought about bodies and minds. But Kafer goes on to craft a "politics of crip futurity," an "insistence on thinking these imagined futures—and hence, these lived presents—differently" (3).

The futurity of Universal Design, while it might also lead to delaying rights and opportunities, makes space for different disability futures that we know are close to impossible to imagine in an ableist society, and particularly in one of its most ableist institutions, the university. The opposite of this disability futurity is "curative time," which entails a "curative imaginary, an understanding of disability that not only expects and assumes intervention but also cannot imagine or comprehend anything other than intervention" (27). These interventions come in service of compulsory able-bodiedness and able-mindedness (27). Curative time is also the time of accommodation—seeking to erase the disability. The potential of UD, on the other hand, is a future with more claiming of disability and a more positive experience of it, not the erasure of disability as some would suggest.

Many of the negative effects of disability can be created by cultural and even spatial constructions—the world is built to accommodate the normal body and mind, and we all experience some degree of discomfort due to these limits. These limits also function to make the world highly inaccessible to people with disabilities—or to make them come in the back door. In response, we could change the environment to minimize the constraining and impairing effects of intellectual and architectural structures, but also to emphasize and enable embodied differences to thrive. Is there a way to increase access without negating the presence of disability? In a sense, this is what Universal Design does—it allows us to claim disability as we limit the normalizing and segregating effects of cultural geographies. For Universal Design to be truly successful, it must do so without claiming to erase embodied difference.

On your own campus, surely there are research initiatives, perhaps highly visible and highly funded, organized around curing disability or eradicating it. These initiatives may not be a problem, per se. But when these initiatives crowd out the space needed to imagine a future in which disability is central and valued rather than eradicated, we badly need a "politics of crip futurity" as Kafer suggests (3). If disability is something we avoid talking about in the push for "wellness" on campus, in creating euphemistic names like "Access Services" or "AccessAbility" instead of disability offices, and if disability is only ever mentioned as something researchers are "fighting," this will undoubtedly impact and negatively shape the environment for disabled students.

As mentioned above, the UD movement was first an architectural movement. The design of physical spaces through UD then also became a means of transforming ideological space. Out of this, Universal Design for Learning (UDL) has become a philosophy of teaching adapted from these architectural roots—advocating the use of multiple and flexible strategies to address the needs of all students. The three major "moves" of UDL mandate that there be multiple means of student engagement (why students learn), multiple means of delivering content (what students learn), and multiple ways for students to express themselves and act (how students learn). In what follows, I will first move backwards, to lay out some of the foundations of UD, and then I will move forward, to acknowledge some of the difficulties of implementing UD in the neoliberal university. But in each of these explorations, I want to center the idea that we must design a future for higher education that acknowledges but rejects its eugenic, steep steps history, refuses to accept an ongoing series of retrofits and slapped-on accommodations, and values instead the unpredictable times and places of disability to come.

Many of the benefits of UD are bound to be unforeseen: the benefits of any design created for a broad range of users will be, almost without exception, unpredictable. So, if we design a product with open-mindedness and inclusiveness, it can have an expanding range of uses. If we design for one body, it will need to be retrofitted to work for any others; if we try to design for all bodies, every single body that interacts with the technology will find a use for it (many of them novel). If we design a classroom activity for one mind (maybe a mind much like our own) then only a few students will be able to do this thinking (students most like us); if we design a classroom activity for a broad range of minds, then all students will have a genuine opportunity to learn and to create new knowledge.

Bringing Disability, Usability, and Universal Design Together

To begin with, there can be no history of UD without an understanding of the history of usability. Allow me to begin with an anecdote. Mara Mills writes powerfully about the history of hearing aids—a technological narrative that every computer science, engineering, and arts scholar or student should read. She suggests that "although the enduring stigmatization of deafness often led to unhappy relationships between individuals and their prosthetics—and sometimes to fraudulence in the hearing aid field—it did not necessarily result in passivity or dependence" (26). So, first of all, much of the frustration that Deaf and hard of hearing people felt was caused by the stigmatization of disability by society, not necessarily by the technologies. Then, these people still went on to play "shaping roles as early adopters, inventors, retailers, and manufacturers of miniaturized components—even though advertisements and the popular press have historically portrayed 'the deaf' as patients, 'guinea pigs,' recipients of charity, or hapless consumers of technology" (26). Mills hits, here, on a key oversight in the history of design and technology: "even in the vast literature on 'users' in technology studies over the past 30 years, people with disabilities have only rarely been ascribed the competence or the relevance to figure centrally in narratives of technological change" (26).[8] Universal Design, then, seeks to change this narrative moving forward; a history of UD also seeks to revise some of these narratives from the past. We begin, then, by revising the history of an interrelated concept: usability.

In their article on the rhetorical concept of "Institutional Critique," mentioned earlier in the book, James Porter et al. wrote about the political move of having usability included as a criteria on Microsoft's "generic product development chart" (610). The initiation of this change proves, to the writers and (hopefully) to the audience, that "though institutions are certainly powerful, they are not monoliths; they are rhetorically constructed human designs (whose power is reinforced by buildings, laws, traditions, and knowledge-making practices) and so are changeable" (611). In their story, getting Microsoft to consider usability was nothing less than a revolution. There are two aspects to this revolution. First, because usability is defined as aiming to "humanize system design," it is an "important political move, establishing users and user-testing as a more integral part of the software development process" (611). The human is set in opposition to the monolithic corporation, and usability seems to be David's slingshot. The second aspect of the revolution is the proof that, because a giant like Microsoft can be changed, even the most monolithic institutions are rhetorically constructed—thus they can be rhetorically reconstructed. It follows that usability itself can be rhetorically reconstructed.

I am particularly interested in the interaction between usability and Universal Design. Usability speaks for universal design, and has played a crucial role in how UD has been rhetorically constructed—and vice versa. In this section, there are two connected theses. First, usability may become a way to talk about user-centered design without always recognizing the diversity of these users—without placing disability at the center of the call for the adaptation of physical, technological, and ideological spaces and interfaces. In the same way, UD has become a way to talk about changing space to accommodate the broadest range of users, yet it consistently overlooks the importance of continued feedback from these users. Therefore, usability needs Universal Design and Universal Design, specifically of education or learning (UDL), needs usability.

Tracing the evolution of the term usability leads directly to its interaction with universal design. The cross-breeding of the two concepts has led to the recombinant terms "Accessible Design" and "Inclusive Design," concepts explained in the book *Countering Design Exclusion: An Introduction to Inclusive Design* by John P. Clarkson and Simeon Keates. Ronald Mace coined the term universal design in a 1985 article in *Designer's West*, and one of the first published articles on UD was titled "Maximizing Usability: The Principles of Universal Design" (Story). This latter article is a primary example of the conjunction of the two concepts, resulting in new sets of principles for the design of physical and ideological space (as well as new portmanteau linguistic products, new words). Given such existent confluence, it seems worthwhile to, at least briefly, provide a genealogy of both usability and UD. I don't intend to give a comprehensive history here. However, I do want to mention some of the commonalities and divergences in the historical development of the two concepts.

Histories

Usability has often been tied to the rights of people with disabilities. Whether in response to a more diverse (and often disabled) workforce following World War II, or in reaction to the increasingly politicized input from people with disabilities about society's barriers, usability foregrounds the ways bodies interact with technologies and environments, and often points out the ways environments and technologies exclude. To trace some of the history of usability we will also trace the circulation of discourse through the body, the bodies that design thinking has selectively excluded, and the bodies that have actively intervened to reshape the world.

The use of more advanced technology in World War II led to a greater concern for the relationship between human and machine. Creating new technologies that had to be immediately utilized by men and women "in the field" led to heightened concern about the interface between person and machine in a life-or-death situation. The ease of this interaction then gradually became a more central priority in the development of new technologies. There was an effort to make machines more responsive to human needs. Following World War II, in North America, the principle of "ease of use" became a key marketing tool—not just for soldiers, or for war veterans (many of whom had different user needs and desires), but for every consumer. Technologies used by people with disabilities—such as prosthetic devices for war-wounded citizens—also were charged with cultural meanings, for instance to mitigate the perceived emasculating effect of injury (access Serlin). Disability, in many ways, came to be seen through new biological, cultural, and technological lenses. At the same time, redesign, with the help of potential users, became a key component of usability theories and methods. For instance, according to company promotional materials,

> As early as the mid-1940s, Kodak created one of the very first in-house corporate design staffs. In 1960, Kodak established what is now one of the oldest Human Factors Labs in the United States. Originally focused on the design of workplace facilities and environments, the lab expanded its charter to include its current focus on product design in the mid-1960s. (Kodak Corp.)

Yet I'd suggest that it wasn't until set principles of usability were adopted in the telecommunications and later in the computer industry in the late 1980s and early 1990s that usability truly became part of the popular lexicon—or part of institutional design in a real and "revolutionary" way. The developments at Microsoft are an excellent example of this change. The key to usability was, and is, the priority of feedback from users—the idea that users must be actively involved in the continued redesign of products, interfaces, and spaces. Central to the development of usability was, simply, the push for more users to be more involved in the design of products. Usability testing represents a shifting of design responsibility—and a sharing of the power that comes from having a stake in making the world—through iterative design. Iterative design, the progressive refinement of design through evaluation by testing actual "end-users" on a working system, brings "the consequences and personal contexts of any knowledge" to light in the early stages of design (Porter et al., 611). Power is shifted to the user who, through use and feedback, can illustrate the ways a technology best fits their needs, tasks, and expectations.

Universal design does not have the same specific history—in some ways, UD developed out of the usability movement. Early discourse about UD borrowed heavily from the discourse of usability. Yet Universal Design is usability with a key difference: it has always been more closely wed to the goal of making the world more accessible for people with disabilities. While usability principles sometimes listed people with disabilities as one key constituency, UD has placed individuals with disabilities at the center. One of the philosophical bases of universal design is that disability is partially socially constructed. Genes alone don't disable people; an environment designed only for people with a certain body disables people whose bodies don't conform to this narrow norm. Changing this environment is a means of intervening in the social construction of disability—interaction between person and world is not only made more efficient, it is made less oppressive. When Ronald Mace and his colleagues at North Carolina State University established the Center for Universal Design in 1989, the associated think tank was named the Center for Accessible Housing, and grew thanks to a grant from the National Institute on Disability and Rehabilitation Research. In 1990, thanks to momentum from the NC State project and other "no-barriers" practitioners, as well as the progressive work of groups like ADAPT,[9] the disability rights movement in the United States made a breakthrough: the U.S. government passed the Americans with Disabilities Act. With the passage of this act, Universal Design gained an essential point for leverage. Previous efforts to prioritize barrier-free design were now given legal reinforcement, and the rights of the disabled user were now inscribed in law. While the ADA hasn't always led to the kind of revolutionary redesign of the environment that we might hope for, it has allowed UD to come in the front door, so to speak—and it has shown how user feedback (in the form of political protest) can create change.

Critiquing Usability and Universal Design

A critique of usability might focus on the failure to prioritize the value of different abilities, needs, and goals in users. As Robert R. Johnson argued in his book *User-Centered Technology: A Rhetorical Theory for Computers and Other Mundane Artifacts*, usability lacks a coherent theory of use or usefulness. Though usability foregrounds the importance of collaboration between users and producers, the ethical foundation of this relationship is underdeveloped.

The ethos of the user most often comes from his or her ability to represent an average consumer or the correct target demographic. Universal design offers a means of placing those with unconventional abilities, needs, and goals at the center of the design process. When disabled people lead the process, we can more specifically address the power imbalances that lead to exclusive spaces, interfaces and pedagogy. On the other hand, a critique of universal design would point out that there is no built-in process for collecting feedback from users, thus no way to ensure that those who inhabit the designed space have an active role in its reconstruction. In these ways, usability and universal design ask for one another. Particularly in the context of the classroom, usability and universal design offer a philosophical and practical basis for the kind of teaching that might be truly responsive to all students, and that might allow all students to be responsible for the direction of pedagogy.

As this communication and expansion happens, then, there is a tension created when we strive to expand toward diversity rather than a normative ideal. As we design pedagogy we must think about the use and usefulness of usability, as Johnson suggests, and we must also consider it ethically. How are particular models and uses exclusive? How does usability, in this way, become a normative process? In an even more specific example, Cynthia Selfe and Richard Selfe wrote:

> [Teachers] who use computers are often involved in establishing and maintaining borders themselves—whether or not they acknowledge or support such a project—and, thus, in contributing to a larger cultural system of differential power that has resulted in the systematic domination and marginalization of certain groups of students, including among them: women, non-whites, and individuals who speak languages other than English. (482)

I would argue that students with disabilities must be added to this list of "certain groups" and that, as Selfe and Selfe argue, they must also be given the opportunity to "become technology critics as well as technology users," to "contribute to technology design," and to "[address] the interested map of reality offered by computer interfaces [by becoming] involved . . . in an ongoing project to revise interfaces as texts" (494–96). Teachers have a responsibility to interrogate all spaces and all interfaces, as well as to share this responsibility equally with our students.

As students and teachers critique spaces and interfaces, lessons from disability studies offer ways to prioritize and to value disability, while developing the critical tools to intervene in the production of cultural space. Disability studies scholarship has had a persistent and insistent, if sometimes neglected or deflected, voice in fields that claim to do the work of design—of spaces or products or technologies. This critical perspective can shed significant light on issues of access and usability. Here, I'll briefly investigate how disability studies reframes issues of normativity, accommodation, and inclusion in ways that must be considered by designers.

As mentioned, disability studies theory holds that disability is partially socially constructed. Disability studies points up the interestedness of categories of disability, and the material and social practices that inscribe, codify, and enforce both normalcy and abnormalcy—the programs and uses of normativity. Disability studies scholars show that disability as an invented category serves primarily to reify or reinforce a fictional norm, organizing classifications of difference around an unexamined, privileged, and normative center. Disability is posed, schematized, and discursively and materially regulated so that dominant positions can be maintained untroubled. The concept of "design against normativity" has even been developed as a response to this maintenance of the norm. As Gesche Joost and Tom Bieling write, "against the background of the cultural construction of normality, the social exclusion of human beings and the design of innovative products . . . majority-oriented design conclusions" cannot be "the guiding principle in usability-focused design approaches" (n.p.). We need to consciously work against the values and habits and biases of mainstream design practices.

So, a disability studies critique reveals something of the normativity of our teaching practices, reflected but also conditioned by the spaces and technologies we engage with. The argument, as it was written by John Dewey nearly 80 years ago, is that "the failure of the adaptation of the material to needs and capacities of individuals may cause an experience to be non-educative quite as much as a failure of an individual to adapt [him/her]self to the material" (47). We also come to understand, through disability studies, how inclusion and accommodation work and do not work, how interested the programs are, and these issues of access and inclusion, then, are crucial for considering the entailments of usability, reframing ideas about who an end user is, how users interact, and to what purpose. Just adding disability accomplishes nothing, and in fact strengthens the squeeze of the norm.

Futures for Disability, Usability, and Universal Design

Universal Design for Learning (UDL) principles focus on multiple, overlapping strategies, not the delivery of single streams of information and not a blanket approach (Bowe). I use the label "Universal Design for Learning" instead of "Universal Design of Instruction" (another way to talk about this concept) because the pedagogy is not solely about instruction; it is about the entire learning process. My definition of UDL, adapted from Bowe, emphasizes expanding three vectors of the classroom dynamic. One focus is on how the teacher instructs—how we deliver information and engage students in the most accessible manner possible. Another focus is on active learning by students—varied forms of applied and interactive learning, with course materials and within a diverse community. The third focus is on multiple options for student design, delivery, and expression— multiple ways for students to show what they know, share their ideas, compose for varying audiences, and then revise. These foci necessitate less teacher dictatorship and greater communal shaping. Universal Design, then, is a way of responding to changing space and developing technology not with panic and reduction but with planning for hybridity and transformation.

As a model, we should consider using the principles of usability in any classroom setting in which we strive for UDL. My 2005 *Disability Studies Quarterly* article makes this argument, and lays out an example of how this can be done: together with students I realized that, although UDL validated and valued their standpoints, there was nothing explicit in the principles of UDL that provided for anonymized student-feedback as part of a dynamic and ongoing, class-by-class process of pedagogy design and revision. Though Frank G. Bowe, in his canonical book-length study of UDL, mentions the need for interaction between teachers and students, this practice has not been codified in a useful way. As mentioned in the previous chapter, the recent work by the New London Group on the concept of "multiliteracies" puts forward a philosophy and a pedagogy of multiple literacies and multimodal learning and expression, and these scholars, including James Paul Gee, Gunther Kress, Bill Cope, and Mary Kalantzis, foreground the role students must be given in the redesign of social futures. Yet the New London Group does not call this universal design, nor do they address learning differences from the perspective of disability. We wanted a more insistent principle of learner negotiation for UDL, based on its principles of inclusion. The students said, repeatedly, that professors would know what works and what needs to be done if they just asked their own students. While recounting a list of strategies that teachers used, and addressing questions about how UDL could be better incorporated, the students continually insisted that teachers had to allow students multiple modes of anonymous course assessment or critique—to give them some control over course design so that their abilities and needs could be adequately addressed as the course went along, not just when it ended.[10]

UD, then, is finally a matter of social justice—the importance of including everyone in the discussions that create space. For UD to be a transformative agenda, we are reminded that our work must be change-enhancing, interactive, contextualized, social; must allow individuals to rewrite institutions through rhetorical action and must push us all to think broadly and generously. Universal design does seem to include, and embrace, such possibilities—and can be beneficially (and continually) rethought when combined with the user-centered and iterative push of usability. Just as usability needs Universal Design, Universal Design needs usability.

We Need to Talk about Universal Design

While I have spent the first half of this chapter arguing for Universal Design, we are required to spend at least as much time arguing against the concept for its potential to come fully into relief, to be totally understandable. We need to talk about Universal Design, and this notion cuts in two directions. First, we need to talk about Universal Design because we need to create more accessible avenues for the presence and participation, creation and collaboration, reading and writing, sketching and moving, revision and reflection of students with a much wider range of abilities and disabilities, levels of preparedness, and cultural and linguistic commitments than we currently do. But, second, we also need to talk or communicate in the sense that something is wrong. "We need to talk" is a phrase that has likely introduced a million breakups. I don't want to break up. But here, I want to suggest that, at the very least, we need to carefully review our relationship with Universal Design. We need to talk about Universal Design. But allow me to clarify that, although we need to talk about Universal Design, it's not you, it's me that has a problem. That is, as you can understand from my arguments above, I have been a longtime proponent of UD and UDL. I have defended UD against those who think it sounds like a variety of creationism or a *Star Trek* episode. I have addressed the doubts of pragmatists and cynics for whom the word universal is understandably, problematically, broad. As mentioned above, I have argued that within the concept of Universal Design we should focus on the verb—design. I have then argued that UD becomes a way to plan, to foresee, to imagine the future. The universal of UD also suggests that disability is something that is always a part of our world and worldview. Thus, when UD is successful, it is hopeful and realistic—allowing teachers to structure space in the broadest possible manner.

As fellow UD proponent and critic Aimi Hamraie has written, the "design" in UD is in fact what Hamraie calls "value-explicit design," design that "does not privilege expert knowledge, but rather provides a framework within which designers can be held accountable for the types of environments that they produce" (n.p.). Thus, the verb "design" in UD also "critiques the false value-neutrality of inaccessible environments" (Hamraie, n.p.). Hamraie cites Edward Steinfeld and Jordana Maisel to suggest as well that the "universal" in UD "be understood as it is used in terms like 'universal suffrage' or 'universal healthcare'" (Steinfeld and Maisel, 30). Hamraie suggests that the "universal" can lead to "broad accessibility"—design for the broadest possible range of users, hopefully considering issues of sex, gender, and intersectionality; aging; size; race, and environmental justice (n.p.). The "universal" can also lead to what Hamraie calls "added value": "designs that produce disability access also have added value or benefit insofar as they are useful to non-disabled people" (n.p.). Though none of these arguments is immune to further critique (from myself or from Hamraie), it is clear that UD can be a powerful lever to challenge the structures and systems that disenfranchise disabled people. It is also clear that UD has been revolutionary within architecture.

This problem of universality is of course connected to normativity. We might suggest that most claims to universality also subsume the possibilities of rich and meaningful particularity. For instance, as Robyn Wiegman suggested, "critical race theorists have assumed that the power of whiteness arises from its appropriation of the universal . . . the universal [as] opposed to and hence devoid of the particular" (117). Yet she argued that, insofar as this assumption is made, "we have failed to interpret the tension between particularity and universality" (117). Wiegman argues that normative and unexamined structures must be rendered particular so that we might understand their power. Likewise, I would argue that we can look for the universal possibilities of particularity. More simply, student learning differences should drive design, should be designed towards.

Importantly, the alternative to planning for diversity is pretty dire, leaving access as an afterthought, situating it as something nice to be done out of a spirit of charity, or as something people with disabilities are being unfairly given. Without Universal Design, the alternatives are the "steep steps" that are set out in front of many people with disabilities, or the "retrofits" that might remove barriers or provide access for disabled people, but do so in ways that physically and ideologically locate disability as either deserving exclusion or as an afterthought.

Posing Problems

As mentioned, despite the "Universal" of UD, there are some major occlusions and oversights built into its implementation. UD has had what Sara Ahmed calls a "melancholic universalism." This can be defined as "the requirement to identify with the universal that repudiates you"— something that a lot of people with disabilities feel about UD, but something that it is very hard to draw attention to ("Melancholic," n.p.). That is, "the universal is the promise of inclusion that has become heavy or weighed down by the way the promise has been sent out and about. . . . the promise of the universal is what conceals the very failure of the universal to be universal" ("Melancholic," n.p.). UD seems like such a good idea that those who might argue against it, or who might point out the ways that it fails to accommodate their needs or minds or bodies, do so only at great cost. Think, for example, of the students who congratulated their teacher on the first day of class for how well-designed the syllabus was, saying that they wouldn't even need the sanctioned accommodations they had been offered. Now imagine what happens when, later in the semester, one of these students feels the need to highlight their exclusion from class, but now must do so against the feelings of their peers and the teacher. As Ahmed writes, "melancholic universalism is another way of describing the promise of happiness; how depression is associated with concrete difference, and how some differences become concrete and not others" ("Melancholic," n.p.). Suitably, she uses the metaphor of a wall (and we might substitute steep steps or ornate gates here, too): the wall "comes up for those who are not accommodated. For those who are accommodated there is no wall at all. Enter; easy, look, easy, just do it" ("Melancholic," n.p.).[11] Later in this chapter, I will attempt to offer some solutions to this exclusion, even as I acknowledge that any solution may be merely a "promise of happiness" that can just as easily disappear. But before we get there, there are more problems.

Interest Convergence

One of the major arguments for UD is that it is good for all students. But of course there is some danger here of falling into what critical race theorists would call interest convergence—the idea that conditions for the minority group improve only once the effort can be justified as helping the majority as well (access Bell). As Brenda Brueggemann and Georgina Kleege point out, for instance, "much of what has always disturbed us about the rhetoric around mainstreaming has to do with the way it is presented as something that is valuable for the *majority* culture . . . culturally enriching non-disabled students" (183, italics mine). In arguing for Universal Design instead of accommodations, many have suggested that UD is of greater benefit to more students—UD can take adaptations and use them to help everyone. Yet such an argument can lead to a situation in which the needs of the majority once again trump the needs of those who have been traditionally excluded—people with disabilities. For instance, here's a statement from the Ohio State FAME website, introducing the concept of UD:

> A key feature of Universal Design is that when you have both ramps and elevators, and even stairs, then you have alternatives even if you don't have a disability. If you're pulling a baby carriage or a shopping cart, you're really glad there's a ramp there, or a curb cut. Or if you've had a large breakfast, you tend not to take the elevator and you

decide, "I'll take the stairs today," but when you're tired, you want the elevator. Options are good for all of us. (n.p.)

While there is nothing inherently wrong with this argument, it does need to be problematized. It is the introduction to UD provided by the section of the site devoted to UD—a section of the site separate from the pages devoted to accommodations. The suggestion is that accommodations may be about students with disabilities, while UD is for everyone. Again, no problem, except that this opens a sort of hole: we can fall into a habit of eliding or overlooking considerations of disability—the power of normativity would pull us toward this elision of oversight. Clearly, having a big breakfast is not the same as having a disability—because most big breakfasts don't lead directly to systemic discrimination.

In response to the interest convergence that situates UD as something that is for "all students," while overlooking specific forms of difference, as well as specific histories of disenfranchisement, a few researchers have begun to explore what might be explicitly built into UD to address the needs, in particular, of African American students. As part of a presentation made at the Pacific Rim Conference on Disabilities in 2006, Higbee et al. presented the following UD principles for multiculturalism and antiracism:

1. Create spaces and programs that foster a sense of community for all students, particularly students from underrepresented communities.
2. Build barrier-free welcoming environments with attention paid to attributes that include disability, diverse content, access to artwork and graphic design, and geographic location relative to function.
3. Design accessible and appropriate physical environments that provide ease of use for people who use different modes of interacting or communicating and allow for confidential use based on the services, programs, or benefits being delivered.
4. Create inclusive and respectful policies and programs that, from the beginning, take into consideration the diverse student and employee populations at the institution and provide natural and cognitive supports to ensure full utilization of programs by students and employees.
5. Hire and develop personnel who understand, respect, and value the institution's diverse community of students and employees.
6. Ensure that nonelectronic information environments are accessible and appropriate so that information is delivered in formats

(e.g., Braille, captioning, different languages) understandable and easily usable by diverse users without requiring unnecessary steps or "hoops" to jump through for completion.

7. Design and maintain Internet and other electronic environments to ensure accessibility and appropriate confidentiality or privacy for those who use various adaptive equipment, hardware (that may vary in age and capacity), and software and for those that require or need confidentiality or privacy (n.p.).

Though some of this guidance overlaps with the usual "list" of UD considerations, there are specific actions here that add crucial dimensions to UD. In particular, the explicit instructions about protecting student privacy really matter. While all students with disabilities may have been (or could be) stigmatized if they disclose a diagnosis, the stakes are absolutely higher for African American students, for whom disability diagnoses and streaming at the K-12 level correlate with overwhelmingly negative outcomes. Racism can and will absolutely compound the stigma of disability. As mentioned previously, ableism is never alone with itself. Keeping any accommodations that are made for these students confidential is a tangible way to avoid inviting racism and ableism. Marking minority students out as those who are visibly in need of a different form of learning might tokenize their involvement and attract other forms of discrimination. As social psychologist Claude Steele has argued the idea: "that erasing stigma improves black achievement [in University] is perhaps the strongest evidence that stigma is what depresses it in the first place. This is no happy realization," but it means that reducing "racial and other vulnerabilities" that come through stigma can improve achievement (6).

Further, in interpreting the extra time and space and "hoops" and "barriers" that minority students may need to navigate, and thus that teachers need to anticipate and build into their course and curriculum design, William Sedlacek suggests that minority students have to develop specific skills and expend considerable energy coping with racism, looking for allies and forming their own community, and protecting their identities (202). It might be argued that these are tasks that might require strategic silence or reticence, cunning, code-switching, self-care, and a wide range of abstract and contextually varying skills. These skills do not always sync with traditional pedagogy and assessment. At the same time, students in "majority" groups can concentrate on interpreting and categorizing information in ways that sync with test-taking, reasoning, and other more straightforward academic arenas (Sedlacek, 202). The result is that multiple studies have shown that minority students, specifically African American and Hispanic students, exert more effort and are more engaged than white peers, but get lower grades (access Greene et al., for instance, on two-year college students and this acknowledged "effort-outcome gap"). Teachers absolutely have to understand that these differences change the social and the educational geography on campus. Universal Design can only hope to address this geography by also imagining a more diverse future.

As Vershawn Young and Frankie Condon have argued, "there are many scholars whose research interests and political commitments coincide with the work of antiracism. It is difficult, however, for even the most committed of us to perceive, name and contend with the ways in which racism winds its way to our classrooms—through unexamined curricula, careless, ill-considered or unreflective teaching practice, or talk to and about our students" (4). Thus there is not a single aspect of the "Universal Design" of teaching that does not need to ask: How might this reinforce the privileges and the exclusions—the steps up and the steps down and the ramps around—the systemic racism of higher education?

Finally, the explicit suggestion to hire or employ diverse faculty becomes a tangible way to remove barriers. It will not be enough to "just" utilize Universal Design in academies where we know the faculty and instructors do not look like and do not come from the same cultural backgrounds as the students. If we do, we are simply retrofitting another academic fad onto a highly exclusive machine. If we make the "interest convergence" argument that UD is just good for all students, we ignore the different pathways that bring students to our classrooms, or keep them from getting there, and we may even reproduce these exclusions.

We Need to Talk about Universal Design in the Neoliberal University

In the last chapter, I suggested that it is likely true that retrofits, in other contexts, can be much more useful and powerful than they can be in higher education, mainly because of the persistence of academic ableism in universities and colleges. Maybe, in the same sense, Universal Design can only do so much in the context of higher education, because of the persistence of both academic ableism and academic ableism-inflected retrofits and defeat devices. That is, disability is so overdetermined by the accommodation process in higher education, and these accommodations can be so efficiently stripped of their effectiveness, that the university is a machine for qualifying (and portioning out only minimal) access and rights.

So we need to talk about Universal Design because despite the potential benefits enumerated above, its usefulness and subversiveness is being slowly vacuumed out. In the neoliberal university, Universal Design may become a way of promising everything while not doing much of anything. I am no longer going to allow Universal Design to make me promises it doesn't intend to keep. Thinking of UD as a logic of neoliberalism specifically can be a useful way to interrogate its meanings, possible uses, and misuses. Neoliberalism takes the values of free choice, flexibility, and deregulation and translates them into market reforms and policies designed to maximize profits, privatize industry, and exploit all available resources. But much more than this, neoliberalism should be seen as a system that powerfully masks inequalities and readily co-opts concepts like diversity, tolerance, and democracy. Not only this, but neoliberalism has been shown to interpellate—to sneak in and insinuate—its logics and grammars into our everyday lives—so that we all become middle managers, so that we run our classrooms and cultural institutions like corporations while allowing corporations to take over the discourses we used to control and sell them back to us for pennies on the dollar. Think of something like critical thinking or information literacy—these are now actual industries tied almost entirely to the creation of a new-economy workforce and having very little to do with their origins in the humanities. I think we are getting dangerously close to allying Universal Design with these same neoliberal trends.

This alliance would place UD closer to what Lauren Berlant calls "cruel optimism"—when something you desire is actually an obstacle to your flourishing; a way of describing how people have remained attached to unachievable fantasies of upward mobility, job security, political and social equality, and durable intimacy—despite evidence that liberal-capitalist societies can no longer be counted on to provide such opportunities for individuals. It is highly possible that a concept such as Universal Design could simply become a proxy system for demanding the flexibility of bodies, increasing the tenuousness of social and physical structures, rebranding our intellectual work, constantly moving the target for technological innovation as flows of information are made ever more proprietary, and placing the privilege of "design" in the hands of a narrowing and exponentially profiting few. More simply, what if we are being given (and we are giving to others) lofty and theoretical concepts like UD to distract us from much more simple realities? What if our debates about the most fair and equitable forms of inclusion are happening as real rights and opportunities get sucked away? UD seems especially prone to the false promise of expanding—neoliberalism promises an expanding world, more jobs, greater access to more and more technology and information. But what expands is truly just the market; this expansion is often false, supplemental, derivative; the benefits of this expansion are only ever financial, they flow upward rapidly, and the benefits that do trickle down do so ever more slowly if they trickle down at all, while risk is transferred downward by the truckload (or pipeline).

It is possible that, in and out of academic circles, the term "neoliberalism" is losing meaning. But it names a relatively simple logic, and a very widespread one. Lisa Duggan suggests that neoliberalism is characterized by the shrinking of the public sphere as the government renounces responsibility for social welfare. This shrinking and shirking connects to a key but misguided concept underlying austerity: the argument that cuts to public programs can lead to private growth. David Harvey has also suggested that the neoliberal state attempts to "reconstruct social solidarities, albeit along different lines . . . in new forms of associationism" ("From Space to Place," 81). In *The House of Difference*, Eva Mackey famously studied Canadian discourses that invoke liberal multicultural practices, but do so in order to protect existing economic and cultural power structures. It is easy to think that a celebration of Universal Design could be a way to actually shrink the safety net and widen structural inequalities. What if Universal Design, as it is being argued for and implemented at colleges universities, just camouflages clawbacks to other essential support systems? These are systems that are stunningly inadequate already.

My warning here is that UD is becoming a neoliberal industry within higher education. While I have offered warnings about the neoliberal dangers of Universal Design in other work, Aimi Hamraie also puts these dangers in stark but brilliant terms: when neoliberal values for UD take over, UD concepts "become marketing tools" and critical discourses "drop out" (n.p.). As David Harvey might say, UD is subject to neoliberal "creative destruction" ("Neoliberalism," 3). This destruction leads to replacing hard-fought provisions with new contractual relations that in fact remove the university or college from responsibility for individual students' rights, and demand that each individual manage their own access. ⟩

I still reserve the right to defend Universal Design. But it also time for an honest appraisal of what our relationship has become. Universal Design, are you a neoliberal buzzword? Have you been creatively destroyed?

Landmarks

In higher education, there are some very tangible examples of the false promise of UD. A recent article in the *Chronicle of Higher Education* profiled a scholar and administrator who had just recently accepted a job as the director of the Institute for Research and Training at Landmark College. Landmark is a two-year institution in Vermont "known for working with students with learning disabilities and ADHD, but now [also] working to understand more of the complex needs of students with multiple disabilities, particularly students with autism-spectrum disorders" (Berrett, n.p.). The scholar talks about the opportunity to implement and then study Universal Design in classrooms at Landmark: "At other institutions where I've worked, it was always a challenge to find enough students to do field research; about 3 percent to 9 percent of the population of postsecondary students has a learning disability. It's different here at Landmark, where all of our 500 students have diagnosed learning disabilities," the scholar said (Berrett, n.p). When Landmark hired neuropsychologist Lynda Katz as their third president in 1994, she transformed Landmark into a research center, thanks to the fact that all students could concurrently be seen as learners and as research subjects (access Toomey and Maguire).

A couple of things to note: first, basic tuition at Landmark costs $48,000 a year. That astronomical number has earned them the distinction of charging the highest tuition of any U.S. college, and they have earned this dubious title every year since 1998. Landmark also ranks 3,152nd in the United States in terms of average faculty salary, and has no tenure process (talk about an economic process designed to extract surplus value with as little investment as possible for the greatest possible return).[12]

Further, the focus of the *Chronicle* interview is not on students, but on this administrator's own research. In the interview, Landmark seems to operate like a laboratory, full of the kind of specimens the scholar can't get at a regular university. A reading of a number of scholarly publications from Landmark faculty, writing about their students, reveals a disturbing trend, characterizing students as having "difficulties with Theory of Mind," using actual article titles like "What's Wrong With That Kid?"

and so on. Landmark also teaches how to teach with Universal Design through expensive online certificate programs, with course titles like "Cerebro-Diversity."

So, what does Landmark stand to gain from this Universal Design research? Hopefully, they improve their teaching. But the research also allows them to market themselves as pedagogically progressive. Doing and studying Universal Design at Landmark reveals a few of the more problematic reasons why we need to talk about Universal Design. First, the very existence of Landmark might signal to teachers in other universities and classrooms that there is a special place where disabled students should go, that they should have to pay a ton to access the accommodations they really need, and, inversely, the "regular" classroom at a "regular" university is thus released of responsibility to accommodate. Or, at the very least, teachers may be allowed to use the excuse that they don't have the resources to do so. This relationship basically exemplifies neoliberalism, where social responsibilities—like the duty to educate all—are left to the open market and paid for by individuals.

But aside from the "special case" of Landmark, more and more programs are popping up at mainstream schools that ask students to pay (usually quite a bit) for accommodations that are labeled as special. At West Virginia University, where I taught for four years, such a program was coming in as I left, and it was called the Mountaineer Academic Program with a mission to "provide student-centered supplemental academic support services for students with disabilities" (Stender, n.p.).[13] There are different levels of tutoring offered, at about $15 an hour. But what happens is that students get funneled to this pay-for-tutoring service immediately, as soon as they come in to Disability Services, and this then ends up replacing what should be happening in the classroom, and also tells teachers that the real accommodations happen elsewhere. The most famous of these programs is Strategic Alternative Learning Techniques (SALT) at Arizona, which costs a lot of money ($2,450 per semester on top of regular tuition), and which offers "alternative accommodations."[14] Such programs, in my mind, answer the minimalistic and harmful logics of the retrofitted accommodation, which uses rights-based arguments against those who are arguing for their rights, but they answer this conundrum by privatizing access and veiling discrimination. This places Universal Design closer to what Lauren Berlant calls "cruel optimism" (as previously discussed). That the flag Landmark is now flying has Universal Design emblazoned across it should give us serious pause.

When these students pay for access and accommodation, they basically sell out their legal rights at the same time as they relinquish their agency, and when this becomes an industry it undercuts the push for equality or diversity across state-sponsored (and privately sponsored) institutions of learning. This isn't to say that separate schools or programs such as Landmark couldn't provide the kinds of access and community missing at many other state-sponsored or mainstream schools—or that students with disabilities should be forced to go to inaccessible schools and fight against their ableist and normative structures. What is happening is much more complex. It is certain that when students with disabilities only pay to enter these special schools and programs, the norms across all universities cannot be feasibly challenged (not that these students have a duty to do so—just that in their absence, teachers and administrators have an excuse to do less, be more ableist). Further, clearly the majority of students with disabilities cannot afford these programs. This all goes to underline the fact that we need to talk about Universal Design.

The Digital Lives of Universal Design

Beyond Landmark and other pay-for-accommodation schools and programs, Universal Design is being used more widely as a marketing tool at contemporary universities. While every mention of Universal Design at North American universities makes claims to validation by citing research, the same very few sources of research are mentioned over and over again, suggesting that while UD initiatives may have begun at places like North Carolina State University, where research into UD was being actively funded, there are very few currently active initiatives funded to continue supporting UD. The same dollars invested in UD back in the early 1990s continue to pay dividends, and no new investment is happening, meaning that UD is the ultimate neoliberal asset: it refuses to die no matter how little is invested in its development or protection.

Using educational-context-specific search tools, for example, shows us that universities that specifically discuss UD somewhere within their web pages refer as well to North Carolina State "about 2,750" times. The linking is significant because NC State is acknowledged as the "birthplace" of UD in their school of architecture. Thus in these 2,750 iterations, Universal Design is likely explained according to its origins. Ohio State is likewise referenced on UD web pages "about 16,900" times and the University of Washington "about 5,860" times. It is safe to say, then, that if an educational website references UD and cites research, that research comes from one of three places: North Carolina State, where the Center for Universal Design's website hasn't been updated since 2008, and where they list no new publications since 2005; the University of Washington, where a series of National Science Foundation and Department of Education grants have funded a series of projects on UD for education; or Ohio State, who received a Department of Education partnership grant to develop UD principles and practices.

The forms of citation of these three projects could be viewed quite loosely: literally hundreds of schools simply reproduce the materials that North Carolina State University, the University of Washington, or Ohio State University developed. For instance, dozens of schools reproduce, in full, Ohio State's FAQs, as Chicago State University does, for instance. This reproduction allows for a nod to UD but certainly guarantees no true understanding or implementation of it, just as students who drag and drop chunks of research into their essays aren't going to be given credit for comprehending, synthesizing, or applying that knowledge. Search for full chunks of text from any of the three main UD hubs and their verbiage appears over and over again. If we need to talk about UD, then we need to ask: Are these UD pages and resources, the vast majority of which have been repurposed and ripped from just three funded initiatives, actually increasing access for students with disabilities, or for "all students"?

Is it possible that having a UD initiative at a school is actually a defeat device? (Recall my definition of the defeat device as a retrofit that is actually designed to hide an inequity or mask a problem by offering a fake or deceiving solution.) That is, could a tiny, negligible investment in UD replace a real investment in more staff, counseling, or other resources? Could a gesture toward UD be a way to say "we don't need to invest in any more accommodations," or even "we eventually won't need accommodations anymore"? It isn't that we wouldn't want higher education to be, eventually, completely Universally Designed. It's just that we are currently nowhere close. So we need to be concerned when we have a Universal Design committee or workshop or conference that is actually encouraging university administrations to invest less in students with disabilities. The same thing might happen through the offloading of UD onto teachers, the vast majority of whom are only tenuously employed. Again, it isn't that we wouldn't want all teachers, eventually, to design their classrooms more accessibly from the start. It is just that, again, we are currently nowhere close.

Checklistification and Neurorhetorics

When colleges and universities present Universal Design on their websites, they sometimes present UD as a list. This listing proceeds from the "nominalization" of UD—its conversion from a verb to a noun, its transformation from a process to a solid thing with clear boundaries, a checklist. The University of Washington's excellent DO-IT project takes this approach, for instance in a "checklist for designing spaces that are welcoming, accessible, and usable" (n.p.). Many, many other colleges and universities have republished this checklist, so much so that it has become a canonical text in the actual academic implementation of UD. But there are some problems with this recycling: How many schools actually use this as a checklist with any teeth, with any consequences? Moreover, turning UD into a checklist defeats so much of the rhetorical purpose of UD, as what I have called a "way to move," or as what Aimi Hamraie has called "a form of activism" (n.p). That is, UD should be registered as action—a patterning of engagement and effort. With this said, such lists invite us to believe that Universal Design would stop if the boxes were all checked. We should be more interested in places to start thinking, doing, acting, and moving.

The one checklist I would be inclined to accept is the simple three-part approach to Universal Design for Learning, as mentioned earlier:

- *Multiple means of representation,* to give learners various ways of acquiring information and knowledge,
- *Multiple means of expression,* to provide learners alternatives for demonstrating what they know,
- *Multiple means of engagement,* to tap into learners' interests, offer appropriate challenges, and increase motivation.

Yet when we begin to break these "multiples" down into short lists of strategies, UDL curls up into a ball or folds up into a small package. The very idea that education is about not just representation but also expression and engagement is somewhat revolutionary in a world of 500-student classes in which lectures and exams are the norm and a course's content is almost always what a textbook or a professor says, rather than what students think or create. Moreover, the "multiple" tells us that there is not just one, nor can there be singular, favored ways of representing, expressing, or engaging—and that is an impetus to view students in a radically broader and more empowering way.

Yet colleges and universities have begun to define UD by linking it with old discourses of "learning styles" and newer "neurorhetorics." So the basic three-part approach, instead of getting opened up to a broader range of possibilities, gets jammed into much more reifying or rigid paradigms. For instance, the "old" idea of learning styles was first used to cajole teachers to move away from an approach to teaching based around a conceptualization of only one type of learner. Stop believing students all learn one way. Stop thinking they will learn the way you do. This was a good thing, and perhaps still radical. But the consequence has often been a labeling and sorting of students: this one is visual, this one auditory, this one kinesthetic, this one a read/write learner. The discourse also linked learning to an innate and fixed student identity—denying the possibility that learning could be social, a process, and so on.[15]

If you Google "universal design" plus "learning style," you'll get all types of charts and images and ideas, and you'll come to understand that advice around UD practices can be pitched to learning styles in ways that exclude all mention of disability. So, teachers can be asked to deliver materials orally and visually, to accommodate different learning styles, rather than to accommodate disability. This gets mapped onto the three-part UD approach: students are seen as specific types of receivers of representation, or they become specific types of expressers, or they are engagers. But this hollows out the potential for disability as a valued and agentive identity in the classroom: Universal Design becomes a way to erase disability altogether. This erasure presents a vexing, inescapable problem for any argument for Universal Design. In my own cautious arguments for UD, I seek to avoid this convergence by urging you to explicitly link teaching/learning strategies to disability experience, when possible, and by placing students with disabilities in the middle of the design process.

A newer flavor of this interest convergence, and this hollowing-out of the activist potential of UD, also comes in the form of what Jordynn Jack would call "neurorhetorics" (n.p.). In this example, colleges and universities have started to pitch UD as something that reaches all parts of the student brain. That is, the three major "moves" of UD now get located in different parts of the mind. In the following chart, taken from a page on the National Center on Universal Design website, but also used by others all over the web, and mainly at educational web addresses, shows how UDL maps across the brain.

The top of the chart is labeled Universal Design for Learning, and

FRAMEWORK AND PRINCIPLES

Affective Networks	Strategic Networks	Recognition Networks
The "why" of learning	The "how" of learning	The "what" of learning

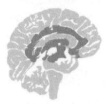 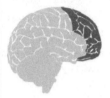 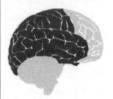

How learners get engaged and stay motivated. How they are challenged, excited, or interested. These are affective dimensions.	Planning and performing tasks. How we organize and express our ideas. Writing an essay or solving a math problem are strategic tasks.	How we gather facts and categorize what we see, hear, and read. Identifying letters, words, or an author's style are recognition tasks.
☑ Stimulate interest and motivation for learning	☑ Differentiate the ways students can express what they know	☑ Present information and content in different ways
Provide Multiple Means of Engagement	**Provide Multiple Means of Action & Expression**	**Provide Multiple Means of Representation**

© CAST 2012, 40 Harvard Mills Square, Suite 3 Wakefield, MA 01880 **Voice:** (781) 245-2212 **TTY:** (781) 245-9320 **Fax:** (781) 245-5212

Fig. 6 "Universal Design for Learning Guidelines." CAST.

this forms a sort of umbrella over the rest of the figure. Below this, we view three columns. The left-hand column is titled Recognition Networks, the "what" of learning. We then are given a two-dimensional side-view of a brain with a region near the back of the brain shaded purple. Below this we can read: "how we gather facts and categorize what we see, hear, and read. Identifying letters, words, or an author's style are recognition tasks." Then there is a shaded box, roughly the same color of purple as the brain shading above, with a check and the imperative to "present information and content in different ways." The center column is titled "Strategic Networks, the 'how' of learning." The brain is shown again, this time with a region near the front shaded blue. Below this we read: "planning and performing tasks. How we organize and express our ideas. Writing an essay or solving a math problem are strategic tasks." Then below this there is a box shaded blue, and another check, now beside the imperative to "differentiate the ways that students can express what they know." The final column, on the right-hand side, is labeled "affective networks, the 'why' of learning." The brain is now shaded green in a circular pattern near its center. Below this we are given the explanation: "how learners get engaged and stay motivated. How they are challenged, excited or interested. These are affective dimensions." The box below this is shaded green, and there is a check, beside which we read the imperative: "stimulate interest and motivation for learning."

This image accompanies the UDL guidelines on the National Center for Universal Design site above—one of the primary pages showcasing the definition of what UD is, in a checklist form. Thus the brains have taken over even the lists.

Other researchers have pointed out how such neurorhetorics (or, in their terms, "neuromyths") have taken over discourse about "learning styles" and "multiple intelligences." As Paul A. Howard-Jones, a neuroscientist writing in the journal *Nature Reviews Neuroscience*, writes, "some longstanding neuromyths are present in products for educators and this has helped them to spread in classrooms across the world. . . . We see new neuromyths on the horizon and old neuromyths arising in new forms . . . and we see confusions about the mind–brain relationship and neural plasticity in discussions about educational investment and learning disorders" (817). The same can be said about the alliance of neuromyths and Universal Design, as viewed in the charts above. Howard-Jones continues:

Multiple Intelligences theory has proved popular with teachers as a welcome argument against intelligence quotient (IQ)-based education. . . . Multiples Intelligences theory claims to be drawn from a range of disciplines, including neuroscience. . . . However, the general processing complexity of the brain makes it unlikely that anything resembling Multiple Intelligences theory can ever be used to describe it, and it seems neither accurate nor useful to reduce the vast range of complex individual differences at neural and cognitive levels to any limited number of capabilities." (818)

As Jack has shown, these charts make what she calls "neuroclaims." That is, they "reduce complex concepts (often subjectivity or identity) to measurable entities in the brain through reduction" (n.p.). This reduction is dangerous first of all because there is really no scientific basis for such claims—no one has actually studied brain activity during Universally Designed teaching, for instance. But within disability studies, we also know that such claims are most often used to infer deficits. As Melanie Yergeau shows, such a scheme "reduces and restricts social forces to grossly simplified, and often binarized, categories . . . renders real human groups passive . . . captives of geometric shapes and other foul representations. The circles, rather than autistics themselves, define what autism is and means. . . . Dichotomizing cognitive styles (e.g., between left and right hemisphere, between visual and spatial)" thus "results in theories of hierarchy rather than theories of difference ("Circle Wars," n.p.).

Erin Manning and Brian Massumi also write that "the neuro is inherently a therapeutic concept contrived with the pathological—which is to say it is guided by an a priori commitment to a presupposed, quantifiable, base-state distinction between the normal and pathological. No matter what kind of philosophical calisthenics are performed around it, the neuron remains profoundly neurotypical" (n.p.). In simpler terms, whenever we are given neuromyths and neurorhetorics, whenever we are given colored brain maps, whenever connections are drawn between types of people, types of thinking, and parts of brains, this is all wrapped up in academic ableism, in ideas about which kinds of brains are normal and the commitment to mark some brains as abnormal, in the desire to place people on steps above and below one another.

If we aren't maxing out all the different ways our brains might be engaged, then our brains are somehow deficient. The same things might be true for pedagogy: once we begin to sew types of teaching to parts of the brain, how do we untangle this from the harm of deficit-based thinking? Once we link the "moves" of UD to discrete parts of the brain, how do we view students as more than just different colors of minds? How do we advocate for critical approaches to teaching beyond the idea of maxing out all modes of teaching, all of the time?

As Christina Cogdell has shown, for decades there has been a "circular approach, whereby a predetermined notion of types affected [physical anthropologists' and psychologists'] selections of groups from which norms were then derived and against which individuals were then measured" (192). The use of "representative 'types' for different population groups [became] a useful tool [not just for] product standardization [but also] 'human engineering'" (192). Against this backdrop, we cannot separate the idea that different people use different parts of their brain from the possibility that this is difference that can be used against individuals and groups.[16]

The good thing is that the original UD materials were designed from the beginning with a great amount of rhetorical velocity—they were always aimed at a common shared audience of students and (especially) educators, and designed to be remixed and repurposed (access Ridolfo and DeVoss). So the FAQ about UD that Chicago State University "borrows" from Ohio State University can do useful rhetorical work in this new location. It could also be said that the discourse of UD helps to change the conversation at universities and colleges. While, predictably, legal phenomena like the ADA is mentioned "about 8,400" times on educational sites that also mention UD, "disability rights" is invoked "about 15,300" times on these pages, and that represents a substantial shift from the legal minima and butt-covering that the ADA seems to inspire, to a rights-based, social justice orientation, one that might even link disability rights to other rights and other linked forms of oppression.

But let's also be realistic. As shown previously, disability services offices are already working above capacity, and may have incentives or restraints, or both, that minimize the supports they can offer and the ways that students might be able to access assistance. Into this mix comes Universal Design: a way to utilize interest convergence to talk about assistance and accommodation without increasing anybody's caseload and without spending a penny.

For instance, McGill University in Canada suggests: "There are several reasons why Universal Design is the model most Higher Education Disability service providers in North America are turning to. These include the need to manage resources of rapidly expanding service demands, building a more sustainable model of service provision . . ." (n.p.). Those "needs" are basically neoliberal justifications for cutting back on funding, not increasing it. So long as Universal Design continues to be gift-wrapped for higher education administrators as something that is more "efficient" and "sustainable," then it will be as dangerous as it is useful.

So, now is the moment in the chapter when I am supposed to offer a much more hopeful message. Now I'm supposed to give everyone some small solution or strategy that we can plug into a problem, at least until next semester.

What I would much rather do would be to give teachers some places to actually begin changing the classroom and the syllabus, without delimiting Universal Design or using it to demand a maxing out of modes, without packaging it as a neurorhetoric or mapping it across the brain.

How do we create change when such change can be so quickly and easily problematized? In his book, *The Rhetoric of Reaction*, Albert O. Hirschman suggests that there are three specific ways that people defuse efforts to create change:

1. The futility thesis holds that nothing we do can have much positive impact at all.

2. The perversity thesis suggests that anything we do to help also creates harm.

3. The jeopardy thesis argues that any change we make will likely endanger something else, something already established, something much more important. (ix)

Each of these "reactions" endangers Universal Design. Of course, they endanger progressive (indeed, all sorts of) political action much more broadly. Further, in terms of the ableism of academia, we know that there are forms of apologia, as well as defeat devices that can always be employed to ignore, defuse, or actually reinforce issues of exclusion and discrimination for disabled people. Hirschman finally argues that there are dangers and risks in both progress and intransigence, action and inaction. The risks of both should be carefully considered, and we need to remember that we can never fully predict the impact of anything we do to create change; but we can know that the futility, perversity, and jeopardy theses, the apologia and defeat devices, will almost always pop up to dissuade people from doing anything at all.

So I present UD not as a grand solution that can be neatly packaged, but in fact as a variety of teaching strategies, each of which might be a good solution in the classroom but might just as well create what Hirschman would call "perversity" or "jeopardy" or what Margaret Price calls "conflicts of access" ("Access" n.p.). That is, the strategy we use to make engagement more accessible for one student could be experienced as profoundly limiting for another. Moreover, often the demand to make a class accessible can be experienced as conflicting with a teacher's access needs. Each of these conflicts should also be seen as a space in which "accesses engage" with one another rather than just colliding, as Dale Katherine Ireland reminds us.[17] This provides an opportunity to rethink the space, time, and infrastructure in which these conflicts arise (n.p.). In a document housed on the University of Michigan Press webpage for this book, then, I offer an exhaustive list of UD "places to start." Teachers can begin with any one of these suggestions, bring them into the classroom, and understand how they meet, collide with, or engage student needs, modes, literacies, styles of learning, and abilities. Any of these strategies may endanger other academic values. But as I have been arguing throughout the book, those values may need to be endangered.

CHAPTER FIVE

Disability on Campus, on Film: Framing the Failures of Higher Education

———— ⚘ ————

Bartleby, the main character from the film *Accepted*, a movie about a college that students create for themselves when they can't get in anywhere else:

"I'm not going to answer your question because I am an expert in rejection." (n.p.)

In this chapter, I am going to discuss disability in popular films that also examine college and university life. We know that disability is generally underrepresented (or suppressed) in college life. But we also know that disability is overdetermined in film. Since the very beginning of its existence as a medium, people with disabilities have been on film and been used as a part of filmic rhetoric. In the famous "Odessa Steps" sequence of *Battleship Potemkin* by Sergei Eisenstein, the presence of disabled people is used to evoke an emotional reaction from the audience. Of course, the steps feature heavily in this scene, too, as the background against which some bodies are shown to be incapable of measuring up. Sally Chivers, Paul Longmore, Nicole Markotic, Michael Northen, and many others have examined the tropes and stereotypes and narrative uses of disability in film, where characters often conform to a series of stock roles and functions. These characters must overcome or compensate for their disability; they need to be killed or cured before the end of the film; they are an "ethical test" for other characters, who establish their likeability and authority and growth in relation to how they treat characters with disabilities; finally, these characters are almost always played by able-bodied actors who receive a disproportionate amount of critical attention and praise for playing disabled. So, let's start with this irony: disability is underrepresented and suppressed on campus, but overdetermined in film, and especially in popular films about college life.

Let's also acknowledge another irony: When I say "popular film" in this chapter, as you'll come to understand, I really mean it. I won't be discussing great films or great art; this is not Sergei Eisenstein. I am going to look to what Judith Halberstam calls "silly archives": archives that allow us to make claims that are remarkably divergent from the claims made about high-culture archives (20). Halberstam studies everything from animated film to *Dude, Where's My Car?* I am working in similar territory here. So, yes, these are not high culture films. I am going to be talking about fairly vulgar comedies like *Animal House, The House Bunny, Back to School, Old School, Accepted,* and *Revenge of the Nerds.* I am going to be talking about '80s movies like *Real Genius* that perhaps can only be framed favorably through the filter of nostalgia. I am also going to talk about a contemporary animated movie, *Monsters University,* that is ostensibly for kids. These have become cult films in collegiate lore. And they are on the Hollywood spin cycle.[1] Yet this is not a "psychotronic" reading of these films, one that ignores political correctness and tries to rescue these films as aesthetic artifacts—in fact, it is the opposite. It is an attempt to engage with the fact that dominant culture has already "ironically elevate[d these] texts that often exhibit a naive disregard for sexism, misogyny" and ableism and transphobia, and on and on (Chibnall, 85). Part of the power of these films is that the dominant culture has already tried to be "psychotronic" about them: saying, basically, we know they are offensive, but let's enjoy them anyhow.[2] Why do we want to treat films about higher learning with such political agnosticism? For my purposes, these "silly" films also offer overt and covert disabled forms of being and acting and knowing, alternative temporalities and economies made possible by alternative corporealities. But I am not here trying to rehabilitate the films or offer an ironic reading of them. College students and the general public still watch these films, repeatedly, and I think educators need to watch them carefully as well.

As Ben Wetherbee argues, we need "a rhetorical perspective on the circulation of images of disability in Hollywood film—a perspective that asks not only if a given movie 'argues' for favorable or unfavorable treatment of marginalized groups like the disabled, but one that also asks how and to what ends disability images function within larger arguments and ideologies" (41). So here's a thesis: these films show, I think, not really a reflection of what happens at universities, but instead disclose some sense of what our culture thinks colleges or universities should be like—and this in turn does influence or frame expectations of what the experience of college or university will be. These are also all powerfully and centrally films about disability, and thus examining these films helps us to understand the inextricable and complicated relationship between higher education and the difference disability makes. Whether the films get disability representation right or wrong may not even be as notable as the fact that, over and over again, when moviegoers consume images of higher education, they are also almost always encountering certain versions of disability.

This chapter, like all of the others, also focuses on rhetorical space. So first I want to examine how films about college and university offer fantasies of segregation: those who are obviously different from the mainstream of college life are physically removed or at a remove from its social and educational spaces in plainly notable ways. As Sara Ahmed points out, "when you realize that the apparently open spaces of academic gatherings are restricted, you notice the restriction: you also notice how those restrictions are either kept out of view or defended if they come into view. . . . to give an account of these defenses is to give an account of how worlds are reproduced" ("On Being Included" 178). Recognizing how groups are excluded from academic life in films—a trope that is so ubiquitous that we might even call it a rule—should show us how readily universities enforce these segregations. These excluded groups do band together. They create new fraternities, for instance. This offers opportunities for new forms of sociality and kinship, yet also underlines the logic of exclusion that is the baseline ethos of higher education. *Animal House, Revenge of the Nerds, Old School, Accepted, Back to School, The House Bunny*, and *Monsters University* all put forward the idea that abnormal or eccentric students can be gathered together, warehoused, and united— and these films cover decades and generations of influence.

Next I will discuss how these films, in justifying the segregation of nonnormative bodies and minds, really reveal the degree to which disability is educationally constructed—created in (perhaps large) part by the administrative, curricular, and pedagogical proclivities and traditions of higher education. How we teach and how we research and how colleges are administered creates disability.

I will then discuss how these segregated or contingent communities develop powerful rhetorics of failure and refusal. These films critique higher education by revealing the unfairness of the supposed meritocracy and by developing alternatives.

Finally, I am going to discuss how the rhetorical structure of these films distills and perhaps even comments on the epistemological nature of disability. More simply, how these films are put together tells us something about learning, about how we learn and about how central disability actually is to this learning.

This chapter address rape and sexual coercion on campus, content that is potentially upsetting and triggering.

Segregating Difference

In these films, we encounter groups with truly, truly diverse populations, perhaps ironically so: for instance *Old School* assigns names like "Spanish" to a Latino character and "Weensie" to a heavyset African American character. In *Revenge of the Nerds* there is Takashi Toshiro playing the Asian stereotype; Arnold Poindexter has a visual impairment; and Lamar Latrell is an effeminate black student. (Takashi dresses up in full indigenous headdress in one segment, perhaps to cover more bases). The nerds also can only be accepted by the black fraternity Lambda Lambda Lambda (who themselves are totally segregated) after they are rejected by all of the others. As Lori Kendall argues, "the film codes the nerds as gay through the fraternity name Lambda Lambda Lambda, referring to the use of the lambda symbol by gay organizations (e.g. Lambda Legal Defense and Education Fund, and the Los Angeles gay pride flag, which includes a lambda symbol)" (269). Further, Lamar "plays a key role in the action, serving in part to code the nerds as all-inclusive. 'We don't discriminate against anyone,' Lewis says pointedly to the national Tri-Lamb leaders" (269). By the third movie in the series, this inclusiveness itself is parodied or ridiculed: the "tour of the Tri- Lamb house early in the movie exposes a multi-cultural, self-sufficient utopia. . . . The film overplays this utopic vision to the point of parody, partially undercutting the presentation of it as desirable" (270). This movie also taps into a sort of badly borrowed civil rights discourse, as the white jocks burn the word "nerds" into the lawn in front of their house. All of this is played off as satirical or humorous, but it belies a reality: as mentioned earlier, minority students have to exert a great amount of energy to navigate racism on campus, working hard to deal with micro-aggressions, for instance, while white students just work hard on their homework. What is a funny ethnic joke for the white characters reveals a true barrier to participation and success for minority students.

The nerds are also shown to be matched up with the "Delta Mu" fraternity, tapping into fat phobia or just plain fat hatred.[3] Booger is the ticking time bomb character, a drug user with violent tendencies, and he even wears a "high on stress" T-shirt and makes suggestions like "we could blow the fuckers up," in response to the threats of the jocks. As soon as the "nerds" arrive they are bullied—the chant of "nerds, nerds, nerds" starts as soon as they step foot on campus. Very quickly, the jocks have physically removed them from the freshman dorm and moved them into a gymnasium—where a series of cots are set up like a refugee camp or hospital. Undesirable students are literally warehoused. The other students in this movie, and in all of the others, are at first constructed as adversaries, are invariably white and good-looking and hyperable. At the very end of the movie, the protagonist Lewis declaims to the student body that "[y]ou might have been called a spaz, or a dork or a geek, any of you who have ever felt stepped on, left out, picked on, put down, whether you think you're a nerd or not, why don't you come down here and join us." His friend Gilbert says: "No one is ever going to be truly free until nerd persecution ends." All of the rest of the students come down and join them except the jocks, who are the real minority. The film ends with the same "nerds, nerds, nerds" chant that welcomed them to campus, but now it is affirmative and celebratory.

Similarly, in *Animal House*, Kent Dorfman—aka Flounder, "a real zero"—is played as intellectually disabled, "fat drunk and stupid." When the outsider group in this film pledges at the jocks' Omega House they get siphoned off into a separate room with other "undesirables": Mohammed, Jugdish, Sidney, and Clayton, a seemingly blind student in a wheelchair. To render this scene, imagine the following film clip: Mohammed, Jugdish, and Sidney are sitting left to right on a brown leather couch. Mohammed wears a white turban and a dark suit and tie. Jugdish looks away from the camera—he has a mustache and is wearing a navy suit. As you can imagine from the names they have been given, Mohammed and Jugdish both have brown skin. Sidney wears large glasses and is the only person smiling. He has white skin and wears a light suit with a sweater vest. Clayton, a white man sitting in a wheelchair on the far right of the scene, wears an olive suit and a yellow shirt. He also wears dark circular glasses and carries a white cane, to visually symbolize his blindness. The filmmakers, clearly, were attempting to cover all of the bases of difference and make it clear that these men were all being segregated from the rest of the party.[4]

The House Bunny offers a fairly uninteresting "flip" of the gender roles, focusing instead on a sorority, as a former *Playboy* bunny becomes the housemother for a group of seemingly "dark" and troubled female students after their previous housemother was "hospitalized with hallucinations." One of these students is pregnant, one talks about her "trailer park in Idaho." The new housemother just turns these girls into sexual objects as they teach her "how to be smart" (so she can land a man). When she says that the fraternity and sorority houses look "like a bunch of little Playboy mansions" she is perhaps far too close to correct, and the sexualized role of the women is something she successfully reinforces. Most female "outsiders" in these films are rehabilitated only once they can stop being such good students and start becoming sexual objects for male students. Thus these films reinforce the rape culture or "sexual coercion" culture on college campuses.[5] I use the term rape culture here carefully. Yet as Jennifer Doyle points out, colleges and universities are run by "communities of men who cannot use the word 'rape' in a conversation" because "always-already there is an agreement not to talk like that" (75). But as I discussed previously, one-fifth to one-quarter of women at U.S. schools will be victims of rape or attempted rape (Fisher et al.); 83 percent of disabled women will be sexually assaulted in their lifetime, a shocking statistic (Krueger et al.); a study by Gwendolyn Francavillo into the experience of Deaf and hard-of-hearing students suggested that 48 percent of these students experienced unwanted sexual contact, at least double the rate of hearing students. In short, rape and sexual assault are themselves a force for disablement on college campuses. And students with disabilities are disproportionately impacted. So I refuse to edit the term out or to discuss universities and colleges without centering the reality of rape culture. These films are artifacts of and promotional materials for this rape culture.

One key aspect of rape culture is that we are invited, asked, or even coerced into laughing at sexual assault—what Donald Trump called "locker-room talk." A rape culture is a culture in which we are told we should be entertained by the availability of women for sex, something that all of these films participate in; they may even lead the conversation. Thus, this sexual objectification is literally a demand—and appropriation into this rape culture becomes the key vector of character development for almost all female characters, monumental and real, and a force for the character development for all male characters, who only become real students through conquest.[6] Acculturation into rape culture is part of the development of outsider male characters as well: in *Revenge of the Nerds*, when the nerds seek revenge for their mistreatment they stage a panty raid on the Pi Delta Psi house and use the distraction to install video cameras to spy on the women while they undress. As the nerds watch these women naked, manipulating the cameras with remote control, the effect is surprisingly unremarkable (though distressing). This camera view is really no different than the filmic gaze upon women in all of these movies, as sexual objects that men go to college to access, discard, trade, or obtain as symbols of status.

One way to be included on campus seems to be to buy into this hyper-heteronormative sexual acquisitiveness. It's what we come across in *The Social Network* when a fictionalized Mark Zuckerberg and his friends create the earliest version of *Facebook*—a panoptical, voyeuristic, and eugenic technology for sorting women based on their sexual desirability. "Facemash," as it was called, asked users to look at two pictures and vote on who was "hotter." The real Zuckerberg, writing on his own blog the night of the site's actual creation, mentioned that "these people have pretty horrendous" images in the Harvard yearbook; "I almost want to put some of these faces next to farm animals and have people vote on which is more attractive" (Hoffman, n.p.).

Of course, the acquisitiveness of many of these movies gives way to the actual hunting of female students in horror movies from the schlocky *Black Christmas* to the *Scream* series. And the fantasy of selection and segregation takes on a different valence in John Singleton's *Higher Learning* and in Spike Lee's *School Daze*, both of which focus on black college life. Amiri Baraka suggested that *School Daze* offers a "'pop' cartoon approach to one segment of black life . . . simply a construction, a composite of scenes to make something like a story, limiting the focus on effects . . . the film presents Black college as a hipper (?), Blacker *Animal House*" (148). Cameron McCarthy et al suggest that "the gangster film has become paradigmatic for black filmic production out of Hollywood. It is fascinating to watch films like Singleton's *Higher Learning* glibly redraw the spatial lines of demarcation of the inner city and the suburbs on to a university town; *Higher Learning* is *Boys 'N the Hood* on campus" (283). Thus, in both movies, the college outsiders are the black students—a trend that is repeated in the recent *Dear Black People*—and this exclusion on college campuses both challenges current exclusions elsewhere in public and political life and reproduces the insider-outsider battles of a long line of college films. What remains constant is the powerful idea that colleges and universities sort students on campus, and sort society more broadly.[7]

In the movie *Accepted*, in which a bunch of high school graduates who haven't been accepted at college create their own university, the segregation is truly literal—they don't make a new fraternity, they create a new school for other "rejects" like them. The inverse image of the college they create is prestigious Harmon College, whose dean opens the film saying: "Do you know what makes Harmon a great college? Rejection. The exclusivity of any university is judged primarily by the number of students it rejects. Unfortunately for the last couple of years we have been unable to match the number of students that Yale, Princeton, or even Stanford rejects, primarily because of our physical limitations. But, all that is about to change. Yale has one, Princeton has one, and now Harmon College will have one: a verdant buffer zone, to keep knowledge in and ignorance out." He wants to extend the Harmon front lawn, literally keeping the rest of the world at a further distance.

The film does a good job of showing that those who are kept out really are a ragtag bunch. The African American character lost his football scholarship when he injured his knee. We have Abernethy Darwin Dunlap who unnecessarily suggests that "you can call me ADD on account of I have ADD." Rory is a stressed-out, overachieving female character. In one scene, the students at this invented college populate their campus with students from an English as a Second Language class that Rory volunteers at when they need it to seem busy. Because Rory also used to "do volunteer work" at the now-condemned Harmon Psychiatric Institute, they also get the brilliantly and profoundly significant idea to rent the old building for their fake school. We watch a montage of the rejected students cleaning up the institution—including bouncing off the padded walls, trying out the electroshock machines and laughing. Later they are shown sitting in the institution's old wheelchairs to play video games or to talk to one another, or wearing the old straitjackets to meditate.

Again, imagine a film still: Abernathy, our "ADD" character, is taking part in a yoga or meditation class. A young red-haired woman sits beside him on the grass outside of a building. We view another student behind the two of them, but this student is partially obscured. Abernathy has blond hair and has his eyes closed. He looks peaceful. He is wearing a white straitjacket, done up so that his hands are pinned against his chest.

When the protagonist, Bartleby, brings his family to campus his sister asks: "Why are there bars on the windows?" He answers, "That's so no one accidentally gets thrown out." Yet this reveals that the bars might be the only difference between this building and a real college building. Notice that the psychiatric hospital is so close to the academy that for Harmon College to expand its front lawn it needs to purchase the property that the hospital was built upon—that shows what the real straitjacket and gown relations have always been between colleges and their surrounding communities. For instance, recall the tunnels connecting my own alma mater, Miami of Ohio, and the Miami Retreat, the asylum just across the street, or the burial sites in Mississippi or Austin I discussed earlier. (I urge you to research the connections in your own area.) The straitjacket scene is played off as a joke and yet, perhaps unintentionally, the setting has the profound effect of reminding the viewer just how tightly yoked together universities and asylums have always been.

We know that people with disabilities have been traditionally seen as objects of study in higher education, rather than as teachers or students. And disability has been a rhetorically produced stigma that could be applied to other marginalized groups to keep them out of the university (and away from access to resources and privileges). The university is also an elite space that justifies the exclusion and warehousing of nonelite and nonstandard bodies and minds in other spaces of incarceration. *Accepted* plays this up as an ironic joke, and yet at the heart of this joke, consciously or not, is an ironic argument about the ways that the rejection, acceptance, and diagnosis of higher education has constructed disability, and has attributed disability to other marginalized groups.

The segregation of nerds and outsiders also has a profoundly eugenic argument to make. Crucially, who partners with whom is a key consideration, and an example of eugenics. That the Sigma Mus—a misfit sorority with a name that is supposed to describe their undesirability—are partnered with the nerds in *Revenge of the Nerds* is also an example of this. Combined with the sexualized role of women in all of these films—women who don't seem to go to class and yet do seem to go to parties—there is a perhaps subconscious, and yet nonetheless profound, eugenic sentiment underlying the fantasy of segregation. These films are about eugenic mergers—a matter I discussed at great length in the first chapter.

Films like *The Rules of Attraction*, *Dear White People*, and *Spring Breakers* paint female students as targets for male professors, with varying degrees of agency in this exchange. Other films like *The Paper Chase* and *Back to School* are really about masculine competition between professors and students for female love interests. Basically, if a college movie isn't about sports, it is about the sport of chasing women. As already mentioned, this reinforces the rape culture on campuses, but it also highlights a eugenic undercurrent: college is about figuring out, often through violent competition, who should mate with whom. This competitive focus on "breeding" is what Francis Galton, the "father of eugenics," called "positive eugenics," something higher education has long had as a key feature: the propagation and mixture of desired groups. In *Real Genius*, which similarly groups nerds and outsiders, Jordan is the "autistic" female character in the film, even though in 1986, when the film was made, we didn't have the same awareness of autism that we now have.[8] Instead, Jordan says that "I am 19 and I am brilliant and I am hyperkinetic so guys are a little afraid, possibly if I stopped to think about it I'd be a little upset." Later, she follows Mitch, a male character, into the men's washroom to say: "I made you a sweater. It's just something I like to do with my hands." Jordan is the object of desire for Mitch, but also an equal partner with the rest of the scientists. She has to partner with another nerd or outsider because no female character in any of these films can avoid being a sexual object. But, importantly, who partners with whom is a key consideration, and an example of "positive" eugenics.

Wherever there is the promotion of the propagation of desired groups, there is policing around the edges of the group. This guarding still happens. Look at the University of Alabama and a recent controversy about sororities refusing to accept African American students—this wasn't just racism and xenophobia and segregation, this was antimiscegenation, and there is a long history of this form of eugenics at North American schools. When we deny students access to the university, or we fail them, we are also cutting them from the supposedly favored gene pool. Sororities and fraternities have long been engines of North American eugenics, and these films reveal how this works. In one profoundly disturbing scene in *Revenge of the Nerds*, a nerd impersonates a jock in the dark to have sex with one of the popular girls. We should find this extremely disturbing because this is rape. The scene also draws symbolism from the trespassing of the boundaries of "positive eugenics"—he is accessing a body that he should not, genetically, have access to.

The eugenic nature of higher education is not a new theme for Hollywood. *College Holiday* is perhaps the most famous film about eugenics to come out of Hollywood—and it is presented as a comic eugenic farce, antieugenics. It's not set on a college campus, but college students are used as "subjects of eugenic experimentation"—in the form of the idealized breeding of desirable students—as Karen A. Keely shows. The film "explicitly ridicules eugenics programs" but "simultaneously and implicitly upholds eugenic ideology" by keeping the unfit from reproducing and showing that the desirable pairs of undergraduates mate up in the end (Keely, 327). All of the films I am studying work within this dynamic to a greater or lesser degree: they reveal the eugenic underpinning of higher education in order to critique elitism, exclusion, and structural inequity, but then most often end up reinforcing these same values across slightly different axes. Real universities were involved in overt eugenic research and teaching and continue to be involved in new forms of eugenic research and teaching. At real universities, structural ableism and coercive sexual culture ensures that "desirable pairs of undergraduates mate up in the end," still.

The different sororities and fraternities in *Monsters University* need to be seen eugenically as well: PNK and EEK, HSS and OK, JOX and ROR. These groups clearly mirror other segregated groups in other college films. There is an undesirable group of women and a clearly desirable group, as well as a scary group; there are men who clearly have the genetic gifts needed to be eugenically desirable, and those who don't. The desired Monster phenotype (or body form) for men seems to be something out of professional wrestling, while the desirable women look like Barbie dolls and the scary girls look like Bratz dolls, and yet both groups are perhaps anatomically impossible. Both are also clearly very physically different from the "EEK" girls, whose name signifies their (un)desirability. Let's remember, as well: this is ostensibly a movie for kids. But the issue is a serious one. As Jennifer Doyle argues, "where we find radical segregation—the complete banishment of sexual difference from a community"—as we do in the sorority and fraternity system in these films—"we will find sexual violence. We will find sexual violence at the center of that world, just as we will find it on its borders" (73).

A final feature of the fantasy of segregation is the sense of real precarity or danger: these students are constantly losing their homes and places to live, there are homeless characters who live in closets, and these movies are peppered from beginning to end with homes exploding or burning down, with people sleeping on lawns or in refugee-camp-like conditions.[9] This insecurity aligns with the fact that there were at least 56,000 homeless college students in the United States in 2015 (Douglas-Gabriel). This insecurity also aligns with Mitchell and Snyder's concept of the "precaritization" of disability under neoliberalism—the ways that "disability serves to identify populations most in danger of rampant social neglect" and expendability (Biopolitics, 19). This highlights the precarity of higher education itself, not just as a game, but as a place where we parcel out life chances from a very finite or small set of real opportunities, and also decide who will be "marked out for wearing out," to quote Lauren Berlant (760).[10] Winning and losing are deeply part of these films—jocks need to be totally vanquished, for instance, and losing often means expulsion.[11] The stakes feel high because this competition has long been built into the college tradition. As Laurence Veysey wrote, the university as it emerged in the United States in the early part of the 20th century "catered to those who sought to compete against men who were basically like themselves" and it fostered ambition to "rise competitively in ways that had been strongly stylized by the urban middle class" (440). The stakes also feel so high because they currently are.[12] Less than two-thirds of college students in the U.S. graduate; 30 percent drop out after the first year; and if you drop out you are twice as likely to be unemployed and you will earn 84 percent less than a graduate (Beckstead).

Through the fantasy of segregation, the characters in these films are, as Aimi Hamraie and Rosemarie Garland-Thomson explain it, "misfit" as they are also "misfits." That is, we actually may rely on universities to mark out and exclude these forms of difference, or to rehabilitate it. I am not at all exaggerating this trend of segregation, and the grouping of physical and mental diversity in these outsider communities—it isn't even a trend, it is the rule in popular films about university. Perhaps the only way to be even more stereotypical is to be totally cartoonish—and that actually happens in *Monsters University* because, of course, it is animated.

The Educational Construction of Disability

Kevin Kiley, writing in *Inside Higher Education*, argues that "more than a comment on college, *Monsters University* is a film about diversity, the innate differences between individuals, and the institutions and situations that help foster connections and understanding between those individuals" (n.p.). Yet it is worth noting that Elizabeth Freeman anticipated *Monsters University* way back in 2005 when the first film *Monsters Incorporated* came out: "the monsters would be right at home on the cover of a corporate brochure or college catalogue. . . . the film presents 'pure,' apolitical difference" because these are all monsters and it is easy to give them a full array of differences in a true spectrum of colors and sizes.[13] *Monsters University*, borrowing the plotline of *Animal House* and *Old School* and other films, is also about a group of outsiders who have been kicked out of an elite program within the university because they don't measure up. Kiley goes on to suggest that the movie is really about "what students in the social and intellectual crucible of college can learn from each other" (n.p.). Kiley argues that *Monsters University* shows that

> a diverse student body adds significantly to the rigor and depth of students' educational experience. Diversity encourages students to question their own assumptions, to test received truths, and to appreciate the spectacular complexity of the modern world. This larger understanding prepares . . . graduates to be active and engaged citizens wrestling with the pressing challenges of the day, to pursue innovation in every field of discovery, and to expand humanity's learning and accomplishment. (n.p.)

This is exactly the sort of organized, normative diversity that Elizabeth Freeman is criticizing in the movie and in higher education more broadly. But despite what Kiley argues, this celebration of diversity is not the message that *Monsters University* finally offers: the two main characters flunk out of the school at the end, and this is preceded by a series of high-stakes trials, rejections, personal risks, and referenda. No matter what the frozen snapshot of diversity is, the protagonists, Sully and Wazowski are marked out for wearing out.

This happens in part because the movie showcases the most diverse possible array of bodies, but doesn't adjust its space at all. The filmmakers studied Ivy League campuses to figure out how to make their animated campus, and then they drop all the monsters in, where they clearly won't fit. Alternatively, we could imagine how these students would push us to imagine a much more accessible campus. A campus designed for learning monsters, so to speak, might be quite a bit better for all students. But this doesn't happen in the film (and doesn't happen, yet, in the real world).[14] This lost opportunity speaks to the idea of "diversity" at all North American colleges—there is some desire for a certain spectrum of bodies but no real structural change to how things are built or how pedagogy unfolds to accommodate these bodies. Monsters University becomes a failure machine.

So these films, in justifying the segregation of nonnormative bodies and minds, also really reveal the degree to which disability is educationally constructed—is created in (perhaps large) part by the administrative, curricular, and pedagogical proclivities and traditions of higher education.[15] All of these characters prove to be disabled by the sociality and the pedagogy of the university.

Imagine two film stills. In the first image, five students are shown sitting in an amphitheater-style lecture hall, diligently writing notes at their desks. But there are also five large, silver, portable cassette players, presumably recording the lecture. The second image appears later in the movie, once all of the students have been replaced by cassette players/recorders. Now, a large reel-to-reel player in positioned on the teacher's desk at the front of the room, presumably playing the lecture. Behind the player, written on the blackboard, are the words "math on tape is hard to follow so: listen carefully."

Recall that I began this book by discussing David Rothman's highly influential book *The Discovery of the Asylum.* The book showed not just how institutions developed, but how they allowed society to impose order through their connections with factories, hospitals, schools, and other institutions (xxv). What is ironic about how Rothman describes asylums and almshouses is that if we were to flip a few key points, we have a great description of the universities also being developed in the same period (the late 19th century): fully removed, rigidly patterned, isolating, labor-intensive, increasingly corrupted and corruptible, but for only the highest orders of society. I argued that perhaps the college or university is in fact exactly the same as the almshouse or asylum, organizationally and even architecturally. And yet we view it as the opposite. Thus the subjects in one total institution, the college, are elevated. The inmates in the other spaces are confined. Importantly: one studies; the other is studied. Films like *Accepted* and *Monsters University,* however, reveal the tightness of the connections between, for instance, prison choreographies and architectures and those of higher education.

As Kieran Healy writes in his brilliant satirical review of the film, "*Monsters University* is a highly traditional institution with many problematic aspects in both its organization and culture. Instruction is resolutely 'chalk and talk,' with faculty members presenting dull lectures to (often very large) classes of obviously disaffected students. Lecture theaters are ill-suited for anything but the most direct sort of instruction" (n.p.). This disconnect is mirrored in *Accepted,* when the protagonist Bartleby sneaks into a class at the prestigious Harmon College and ends up in a "spillover" room listening to a lecture from a speaker perched on the lectern, or in *Back to School* when Rodney Dangerfield's character sends his secretary to take notes in all of his classes, or through a running joke in *Real Genius* wherein students begin leaving tape-recorders in their seats in a class and we witness the room filling with more and more tape recorders as the semester progresses, until the lecturer is also now replaced by a tape player and the room has only tape recorders and no students. This could be read as a prescient argument—a good prediction—about the ways higher education might be undermined by online learning and other pedagogical innovations in the near future, and Healy makes this point, but I read this as a critique of the normative pedagogies, the dominant and traditional ways of teaching in these schools. Even though *Real Genius* was made in the mideighties, it can still be read as a critique of the ways that rote learning, memorization, attendance, listening, duplicating, and other modes are overemphasized, while teachers are undersupported, facilities are subpar and inaccessible, and so on.

Yet in contrast to this seeming "checking out" of students, consider all of the ways that participation is now mandated in higher education. Bruce MacFarlane, writing in the *Times Higher Education* supplement in the United Kingdom, points out how "lecturers elicit responses from students in class by calling on individuals to answer questions or give an opinion. The use of clickers, hailed as an 'innovative' practice across the sector, has much the same effect. This enforced participation contrasts starkly with the way academics treat each other at conferences, where we generally grant our peers the right to reticence" (n.p).

In classroom scenes in all of these movies, professors channel power through the fact that they can call on any student, at any time, and test their knowledge on the spot. This is the opposite of my universally designed note-card activity, played out over and over. MacFarlane's essay goes on to call attention to many other spheres in which the freedom that scholars enjoy is not passed along to their students. For instance, "there are now strict rules on attendance at many university classes and growing use of 'class participation' grades as a means of rewarding so-called student engagement. These are reliant almost entirely on crude indicators, such as turning up or asking questions, rather than harder-to-observe measures of genuine learning" (n.p.). Margaret Price's work on the ableist nature of these participation measures is crucial to mention here, too (access Mad at School). MacFarlane argues that "such compulsory attendance rules represent an intergenerational hypocrisy, since they have been developed and implemented by baby boomers who were never subject to such restrictions on their own academic freedom" and now academics who "jealously guard our own academic freedom" fail to understand "enough about why student academic freedom is so important" (n.p.).

Most of these movies about higher education reveal that when we take classes in which memorizing class content and then being tested on it is central, and add mandatory participation, we get a class full not of tape recorders, but full of students using mainly the aspects of their intellect that best allow them to memorize and to perform normative gestures of participation.

In the films, most often we view large groups of students acquiescing to these strange educational demands. Yet the films need to portray to the audience what the toll of these normative pedagogies and processes actually is. So there is also a "ticking time bomb" character in nearly all of these films. We might classify this student as a third type of Samantha: Scary Samantha. In *Back to School* this character is played by a Vietnam veteran professor who is described as "really committed or I think he was"—and constructed as having post-traumatic stress disorder (PTSD). In another scene in which students are studying in a library, a student simply jumps up and begins screaming and runs out of the room. In *Accepted*, the elite Harmon College is accused of "putting so much pressure on kids that they turn into stress cases and caffeine freaks . . . you rob kids of their creativity and passion." Clearly, characters are given mental or psychological disabilities as markers of their difference, and yet the university environment is also shown to make professors and students "crack" or go "crazy."

We witness a troubling binary between the expectation that these outsider students have to be geniuses (overcoming and compensating for their disability or difference) and a fine line between genius and violence, a trope that we are seeing more and more in higher education post–Virginia Tech, or even post–Umpqua Community College. The "ticking time bomb" character in *Accepted*, when asked what he wants to learn says, darkly, "I want to blow things up with my mind." The film ends with him seemingly using this power to blow up the BMW of the dean of Harmon. The scene may have been intended to be played for laughs, but it is hard to view as anything but quite scary. *Real Genius* ends with the outsiders aiming a laser at a professor's house and using it to fill the mansion with popcorn, a much less threatening gesture but nonetheless a troubling statement about the tight binary between extraordinary and nonnormative intelligence and the societal belief that the flip side of thinking differently is the potential for acts of aggression.

On the other hand, Katie Rose Guest Pryal writes about the trope of "creativity mystique," wherein mood disorders are correlated with creativity. This trope is "a product of the era of modern psychiatry, [and] suggests not only that mood disorders are sources of creative genius, but also that medical treatment should take patient creativity into account" (n.p.). Pryal shows how conservative scientific literature has begun to draw that correlation, but also how more fringe scientific and pop-scientific publications have begun to go so far as to suggest a causal link between mood disorders and creativity, or even "inverse-causation" wherein creativity causes mood disorders (n.p.). This research may greatly affect treatment options, but it also constructs mood disorders as phenomena that had better connect to genius. Emily Martin, in *Bipolar Expeditions*, also suggests that as we begin to understand manic depression as an "asset," we may be constructing two kinds of mania: a "good" kind characterized by successful celebrities and a "bad" variety "to which most sufferers of manic depression are relegated" (220). The consequence is that "even if the value given to the irrational experience of mania increases, validity would yet again be denied to the 'mentally ill,' and in fact their stigmatization might increase" (220). In these films, we recognize both treatments: "real" geniuses fabricated by the creativity mystique, and ticking time bombs. We would be well advised to think carefully about the roots of both of these tropes in films about collegiate life. Both tropes, after all, do very little to shift the focus to the ways that disability is educationally constructed. Which students (from which backgrounds, and under which circumstances) get to be geniuses, and which drop out, for example, and why?

Because we should note also that in almost every single one of these movies the climactic scenes involve some form of extremely high-stakes testing—most often involving a mixture of sporting events, perhaps some drinking, and more traditional scholastic contests like debates or speeches. In almost all of these climactic sequences, the outsiders compete well but eventually lose. They are clearly adapting themselves to events for which they are not ideally suited, unlike their jock competitors, and the triumph is that they even hold their own. But there are clear winners and losers, without a doubt. This trend needs to be twisted into some form of critique of the adversarial, normative, very physically demanding, very time-sensitive and urgent, very high-stakes nature of the entire curriculum and pedagogy of the university.

As Tanya Titchkosky argues, "there is an intimate relationship between establishing disability as an important form of critical knowledge production within the university and creating accessible learning environments where learning communities can thrive" (70). Yet these movies, while they feature a wide arrange of bodies, disabilities, and learning "styles," rarely argue that the pedagogical or physical architecture of the schools should be made to accommodate, let alone transform. Whereas audio recorders could in fact add to the accessibility of a classroom, they serve to undermine the value of the version of education put forward in these films.

As Healy writes in his satirical review of *Monsters University*, "Classroom spaces also seem poorly equipped to address the needs of nontraditional monsters, especially giant monsters. . . . all of the classrooms are tiny, or accessible only by very small doors that even a moderately-sized undergraduate would have trouble fitting through" (n.p). Disturbingly, the two most giant monsters are both depicted playing sports: a female giant monster is shown playing giant ultimate Frisbee (or possibly ultimate giant Frisbee), and a giant slug monster is evidently the key player on the football team.[16] Healy's review gets at a key feature of each and every one of these films: the educational/architectural construction of disability.

Here we would also do well to recall some numbers I have mentioned a few times already: the average annual disability services office budget in 2008 was $257,289 (Harbour, 41). These are the places where students are supposed to be able to access the means of countering those structures and processes that disable or that create an uneven playing field. Yet this budget is equivalent to the average salary of a single dean like Monsters University's Dean Hardscrabble. And we know that more and more services at colleges and universities are being offered as pay for accommodation and framed as outside of the usual role of the disability services office. Characters do critique these constructions, as when Robert Downey Jr.'s character in *Back to School* mounts a pseudo-Marxist critique of the university as a machine for capitalism, yet this is undermined when Downey's Marxism is shown to be focused on remedying unequal access to women.[17] So, while these films do propose changes, too often the changes are hyperbolically revolutionary, not incremental or practical.

Perhaps Lewis Black's Dean Lewis in *Accepted* puts it best: "Look, we throw a lot of fancy words in front of these kids in order to attract them to go to school in the belief that they are gonna have a better life. And we all know what we are doing is breeding a whole new generation of buyers and sellers . . . and indoctrinating them into a lifelong hell of debt and indecision." *Accepted*, through this alternative college set at an old psychiatric hospital, and as the clear exception to the other films' academic ableism, does begin to develop the curriculum and pedagogy to challenge the ways in which mainstream colleges and universities construct disability and portion out life chances.

Failure and Refusal

This leads me to my next point: these segregated or contingent communities develop powerful rhetorics of failure and refusal. These films can be seen to critique higher education by revealing the unfairness of the meritocracy and by developing alternatives.[18] This has been a theme throughout this book and throughout history. From the disabled students movement at Berkeley (certainly as well as before it), to examples like Navi Dhanota's successful human rights complaint in Canada, to the #academicableism campaign in the United Kingdom, to the ongoing activist work of disability studies scholars like Sam Schalk, Catherine Kudlick, Melanie Yergeau, Sara Maria Acevedo, or Margaret Price doing coalitional work for various forms of access, to local organizations like Students for Barrier-Free Access at the University of Toronto, to the students with disabilities on your own campus navigating and negotiating attitudes and structures every day, there has always been resistance to academic ableism. So we shouldn't be surprised that these movies center on themes of student solidarity and defiance.

Monsters University, Old School, Back to School, and *Real Genius* are all driven by the prospect of the protagonists either flunking out of school or of being rejected. But by the time the movies end we understand that the success that higher education offers isn't worth all the trouble. Their eventual failure doesn't stop the characters from jumping through all of the hoops and measurements necessary to be deemed successful under these ridiculous terms; it just stops them from finally accepting the idea of being judged by them. Thus we have a critique of the system without assimilation into the system; yet we also have a capitulation or bending to every measure of the system before it is finally rejected. These refusals are often shadowed by critiques of capitalism, and yet most often are resolved with failures in academia that instead often serve to advance the cause of capitalism, entrepreneurialism, and bootstrapping. I've been writing, after all, about the ways that academia structures and creates disability, and through the climactic high-stakes contests in these films the outsider groups show themselves capable of competing on this very normative stage.[19] But they don't succeed. Often, they choose not to.

Monsters University ends with Sully and Wazowski dropping out of school and getting mailroom jobs instead.[20] In *Accepted*, the entire film is premised on failure, and Bartleby, whose name is no accident, turns this failure into an art—or into Arts and Sciences. As Scott Sandage writes, "Black and white are the favorite colors of capitalism, which pays a premium for clear distinctions and bold contrasts. Failure is gray, smudging whatever it touches. However unsightly, failure pervades the cultural history of capitalism" (10). He goes on to argue that "American capitalism has been constructed so that we see failure as a 'moral sieve' that trap[s] the loafer and pass[es] the true man [*sic*] through" (17). Clearly, we are asked to understand the North American university as very much a central part of this moral sieve. Yet failure can have its own moral or ethical subversiveness.

Bartleby is also the name of Herman Melville's protagonist, famous for refusing to do the work—mindless copying and writing—that is asked of him. He is one of the most famous refusers in literary history—and it is no coincidence that the main character in *Accepted* is named Bartleby. As Gilles Deleuze says of Melville's character: "Bartleby is neither a metaphor for the writer nor the symbol of anything whatsoever. It is a violently comical text, and the comical is always literal" (76). As mentioned, many of these films are driven by the prospect of the protagonists either flunking out of school or of being rejected. But by the time the movies end we are led to believe that the success that higher education offers isn't worth all the trouble. *Accepted* flips the script by setting up an entirely alternative university without accreditation.

Once Bartleby realizes that thousands of fellow rejects have now enrolled at the school he created as a lark, he simply asks them what they want to learn. Most of the men say "girls,"[21] yet others choose and then create classes like "getting lost," "walking down the road thinking about stuff," "doing nothing," "dreaming," and "bullshitting." Like Universally Designed classes, these seem to allow a lot of tolerance for error, positive redundancy, and true choice of modes of engagement (and disengagement). "The students are the teachers" at the South Harmon Institute of Technology (SHIT), and they call themselves SHITheads.[22] Much like the argument for UD, the SHIT curriculum is based in the idea that normal and normate pedagogy are ineffective, and specifically out of touch with the ways that a diverse range of bodies might learn.

In front of a state review panel at the climax of the movie, Bartleby says "I'm not going to answer your question because I am an expert in rejection and I can see it in your faces. . . . We came here today and ask for your approval and something just occurred to me, who gives a shit." Likewise, Blutarski's famous speech in *Animal House* calls for "a really stupid and futile gesture." In *Real Genius*, instead of allowing an evil professor to use their laser for military purposes, the outsiders use it to microwave a massive amount of popcorn, which they eat in slow motion as Tears for Fears' "Everybody Wants to Rule the World" plays in the scene that ends the movie.

As Lisa Le Feuvre writes, "Failure, by definition, takes us beyond assumptions about what we think we know" and "the embrace of failure can become an act of bravery, of daring to go beyond normal practices and enter a realm of not-knowing" (13). Judith Halberstam explains that "as a practice, failure recognizes that alternatives are embedded already in the dominant and that power is never total or consistent" (88). This exploitation also offers clear resonance with disability studies theory. Halberstam argues that "while failure certainly comes accompanied by a host of negative affects, such as disappointment, disillusionment, and despair, it also provides the opportunity to" critique the belief that "success happens to good people and failure is just a consequence of a bad attitude rather than structural conditions" (3). She argues that "under certain circumstances failing, losing, forgetting, unmaking, undoing, unbecoming, not knowing may in fact offer more creative, more cooperative, more surprising ways of being in the world" (2–3). Failure can reveal structural ableism and other forms of entrenched oppression while making space for other ways of knowing and learning. This is clearly the argument that *Accepted* in particular is making, yet all of these movies to a certain degree champion failure as a means of critiquing the disabling structures and the false meritocracy of higher education.[23]

In *Accepted*, Bartleby's father argues that "Society has rules. . . . if you want a happy and successful life, you go to college." Yet, after getting expelled from Monsters University, Mike and Sulley manage to achieve success without earning their degrees, by working their way up the bureaucracy at Monsters Inc., allowing Kiley to suggest that this "plays into the popular zeitgeist that questions the value of a college degree, reinforced with the Gateses and Jobses and Zuckerbergs that have captured public imagination. But it is an ending that certainly runs counter to the data" (n.p.). In *Back to School*, Thornton Melon is a self-made man (owning a chain of Tall & Fat clothing stores) but what he lacks is taste and class. He buys his way into college by paying for a new business school building. Dean Barbe then suggests that "Mr. Melon thinks he can buy his way out of the gutter." Melon replies: "While you were tucked away up here . . . I was out there busting my hump in the real world. . . . the reason guys like you have a place to teach is because guys like me donate buildings" (n.p.). Later, in the bookstore, literalizing this relationship, he foots a giant bill for his fellow students: "It's on me, Shakespeare for everyone" (n.p.). This calls to mind my earlier discussions of the economics of higher education, and the influence of academic investments and giving—where the very genetics of the student body are intentionally shaped by the potential of students to become benefactors.

These acts of failure and of corruption are often infused with powerful anti-intellectual sentiment. But why do we want to view stories in which college degrees can be bought, or in which they aren't worth anything at all? Perhaps these sentiments reveal how disability studies' critiques of the inaccessibility of higher education can and cannot engage with larger societal critiques of the academy.[24] In simpler terms, what if the general public would be completely unsurprised to hear about the ableism of the academy because higher education is something they've distrusted from the word go? These films construct one group of students as "rich and lazy" or "privileged, because school is a luxury" and on the other hand they construct another group of students as "poor, naïve and foolish" until they realize that college is something they cannot afford or should not invest in (Doyle, 115). There is very little room between these two extremes. So these films seem to show that popular culture doesn't trust college or university very much, in part perhaps because the outsiders or underdogs are so clearly disadvantaged by its normative cultures and mechanisms, even if the "real world" is no less ableist.

The films also make real what Mitchell and Snyder call "a nonnormative positivist approach" in which the failure and refusal of outsiders, and particularly disabled students, represent "modes of recognition" that "facilitate the mutating potentials of life in the interstitial social alternative of crip/queer socialities and collective consciousness" (Biopolitics, 114). Much more simply: when we even witness disability on campus, on film, this challenges the normativity of film and of campuses. Even if these alternative roles and oppositional stances can be easily coopted, they do open up the possibility of a differently embodied position and a different attitude toward school. This might be metaphorized by the title *Back to School*, a title that also narrates a positionality: turning one's back on school or, at least, approaching it sideways, skeptically. This is an apt description of general public sentiment about university and college life and learning.

But who is this "public"? It seems that some of the popularity of this critique is generational. If you can laugh at higher education as a college graduate, it may allow you to reinforce the sense that the hoops you had to jump through were more difficult, and the merit you've received and privilege you have access to are thus more deserved than those of "kids these days." If you didn't go to college and don't plan to, the critique is also about reinforcing the systems and beliefs that assign value to your own (different) path and your own (different) choices. In a culture in which higher education seems like a monolithic "good" and a require- ment for access to privilege, it is reasonable to want to critique it and valorize other options—maybe this is why we celebrate some of these characters dropping out.

In the end, watching these films might convince us that the public doesn't seem to like university administrators or professors, and also seems to dislike the students for whom success in their university studies seems natural and easy. In a climate in which academia is increasingly under fire for "coddling" students, for promoting identity politics, for being too "liberal," it will be increasingly important to better understand these critiques and this "back to school" positioning.

The Disabled Professor: How to Win an Oscar

Hollywood (and the broader public) may have its back to school, and this may or may not be useful for creating a larger critique of education. Yet, on the other hand, Hollywood seems to love disabled professors. Eddie Redmayne won an Oscar in 2015 for his portrayal of Stephen Hawking in *The Theory of Everything*. Julianne Moore also won for her portrayal of a professor with early-onset Alzheimer's in *Still Alice*. From *A Beautiful Mind* and *Temple Grandin* to these recent examples, it's a long-held act- ing truth: Want an Oscar? Go disabled. The argument goes that an actor playing a disabled character is stretching their theatrical chops, because disability has to feel like the most foreign experience there is. When that able-bodied actor confidently walks up to the stage to eloquently accept their Academy Award, everyone can feel better knowing that it was all an act. Redmayne and Moore used their Oscar speeches to raise awareness of ALS (Amyotrophic Lateral Sclerosis) and Alzheimer's, respectively. Redmayne even said his award was "for all those people battling ALS." Yet Moore joked that winning an Oscar is supposed to make people live five years longer, reminding us that she is not *Still Alice* at all. And that's important: because the audience is supposed to feel that they too are not Alice, and not Stephen Hawking.

Further, in movies in which a character becomes progressively more disabled, as happens in both *The Theory of Everything* and *Still Alice*, having an able-bodied actor to flash back to throughout the movie strongly reinforces the idea that the able self is the real person underneath the disability. Disability is just a neat costume. We're encouraged to identify with the able professor they were, rather than the disabled person they've become (and the disabled people we will all become). The movies thus play on the fears of many temporarily able-bodied academics: What if the very things that I have based my career around—my intellect, my ability to concentrate, to "stand and deliver"—were gone tomorrow? This fear overwhelms much more reasonable questions, like, for instance, what will my employer do to protect my right to workplace accommodations as my abilities change, because all abilities do? What can I do to advocate for the rights of others who can contribute to academia greatly, but need a few accommodations to do so? *Still Alice* and *The Theory of Everything* might just succeed in Hollywood because they do not lead anyone to ask such questions.

In these films, when a medical professional explains the character primarily through their deficits and diagnoses, the audience is supposed to feel scared. In Moore's case, Alice's role as a scholar adds to the power of this diagnosis. We are supposed to feel pity because the expert is now the specimen. This pity might, ideally, reveal some of the power imbalance of medicalization, or the ways that higher education reinforces the binary between researcher and researched, medical authority and medical anomaly. But in Hollywood, more often it simply robs the disabled person of agency, renders them powerless, and makes their identity mainly about the disability.

As mentioned previously, in Canada, there are barely more than 200 professionals employed to provide disability accommodations at colleges and universities. In the United States, the average operating budget of an entire disability services office is about $250,000. That could pay for one-eighth of a college football coach, or for the dress that Karl Lagerfeld made for Julianne Moore to wear at the Academy Awards. This lack of investment tells the rest of the university that disability doesn't matter. But watch *The Theory of Everything*, and you can retain the fantasy that all students and faculty with disabilities get accessible housing and technology, that they might even get star treatment, and that they are sure to succeed if they keep working hard.

Of course, in *Still Alice*, we do get a harsh and realistic reminder of what disability can mean in the real world: when Alice discloses her disability to her department chair at Columbia University, she is almost instantly fired. Please don't think that what happened to Alice in the film was either legal or ethical. It wasn't. The trope of the disabled professor should at the very least reveal that people with disabilities can and should work in any career, including higher education. That means that they can't just be fired for disclosing their disabilities. But that also means that Hollywood could do a bit more to reveal the fact that, Stephen Hawking and Temple Grandin aside, students and faculty with disabilities are much more likely to experience the stigma and mistreatment Alice receives than the star treatment Hawking does. In the real world, academics with disabilities could all be supported as Hawking is, but most are mistreated as Alice is.

As a star researcher, and a tenured worker, Alice would have had protections that the vast majority of teachers in higher education do not have. And many faculty members fear that requesting accommodation of any kind will be seen as a sign of weakness or inability to perform, particularly in a neoliberal climate that demands hyper-productivity and individual flexibility from all members. When Margaret Price published "It Shouldn't Be So Hard" in *Inside Higher Ed* in 2011, arguing for a more accessible climate for disabled faculty, for example, numerous responses to the essay only reinforced the sense that faculty members should mask or carefully disguise any weakness or inability to perform. For instance, one commenter wrote, "In today's job market, when there are well over a hundred qualified applicants for a tenure track position, there is little basis for hiring a person who will struggle with half of his or her job duties." Another added:

> I'm sorry but some of these things (it differs for everyone) that are required to be a professor are hard. It comes with the territory so we don't go head first into the realm of snowflakes and gumdrop unicorns. . . . As much as you want it to be an issue of diversity it is not. It is about the work load in a department and our interest in hiring someone who will do it effectively. (n.p.)

Not much has changed in the intervening semesters since 2011. In spite of some calls for faculty to be more open about disability, the administrative and cultural milieu for disabled faculty remains relatively inhospitable, whether overtly or covertly. It's still very, very hard.

Disabled people with PhDs are much more likely to end up underemployed, exploited as adjunct labor, and to experience discrimination as a result of their disability. A 2012 study published in the journal *Work* found that 15% "of faculty and staff respondents were found to have disabilities, with 26% reporting experience of job discrimination, and 20% reporting harassment because of their disability" (560). As the *Inside Higher Ed* commenters highlight, faculty attitudes about disability seem to sort their potential colleagues into two fictional worlds: the world of the superhero (like Hawking), where that disabled colleague will dramatically compensate for their disability, rising above the competition, or they will exist in the world of "gumdrop unicorns," where asking for the right to accommodation, a right established a quarter of a century ago in the United States, situates you in a fantasy world.

So, why do disabled characters show up in Oscar nominations year after year, yet with no disabled people in these roles? Well, Hollywood is in this way just like higher education, where disability is studied and represented everywhere, most often in the absence of the employment of actual people with disabilities, and definitely in an environment in which it is still profoundly dangerous to disclose disability. Hollywood thus ensures that the public never really understands disability as a culture or a movement, never views disabled people as the largest minority in North America, with rights that are often unprotected and overlooked. The Academy also ignores the tremendous artistic—and academic—production and talent of disabled people themselves. Disability can safely continue to exist as something purely theatrical and highly theoretical.

Not Yet

In *Still Alice*, a key scene involves Moore running around her campus—jogging for fitness. Though it seems clear that Alice has run this route thousands of times, that she is fully "at home" on this campus, that this "wellness" or "mental health" regime has long been a key part of her academic day, in this scene she becomes confused, can't recognize where she is. On her own campus, she is all of a sudden totally lost. This is supposed to be upsetting, and signal that something is not right with her brain. At the beginning of *Monsters University*, we view a slug slowly making their way to class—an example of a Slow Samantha, it would seem. At the very end of the movie, after what we are to suppose is a full year or at least a full semester of school, the slug finally makes it to class. This is supposed to be funny. But there is much we can learn from the slug, and from Alice. Finally, I am going to discuss how the rhetorical structure of these films distills and perhaps even comments on the epistemological nature of disability—or the ways that disability might help us to think and move through higher education differently.

First, I think we can understand that the slug represents what Tanya Titchkosky calls the "not yet" time of disability within higher education: there is no way that the environment is going to accommodate his pace individually, but his trajectory also physicalizes the chronology of being "marked out for wearing out" in higher education, or the ways that college keeps certain bodies and minds in abeyance. The slug is moving in what we can call "crip time": "recognizing how expectations of how long things should take account [of a range of] types of minds and bodies" so that we can "bend the clock" rather than bending bodies (Kafer). Margaret Price suggests that crip time is the "flexible approach to normative time frames" (62). Crip time has generally been interpreted as responsive: a way to impose critical delay through the refusal to follow strict schedules (schedules that might be normative, ableist, medically rehabilitative, and so on). Time marches on, and we can refuse to roll with it. But in arguing that a standard and obedient response to time and timing actually overlooks unique opportunities for making meaning, we can also situate crip time as an epistemology—a way of thinking and moving.

Normative time, on the other hand, is what usually structures college life. Recall for instance the parallels between the tight scheduling of the asylum and that of the university, from Rothman's history, or the parallels between the "eugenic design" of factories and of a version of higher education that was intended to produce factory workers. Normative time renders the slug late, rather than the college campus inaccessible because it doesn't have a bus for slugs. Normative time renders Moore not just lost, but panicking and checking her watch because she is also suddenly late. And curative time, as Kafer has shown, syncs with this normative time because it describes the patterns in which one must always be getting better on a college campus, which is why going for a jog seems like such a perfectly academic thing for Moore to do.

On the other hand, crip timetabling happens in *Accepted* when students ask for classes like "getting lost," "thinking about stuff," "doing nothing," or "dreaming." These are subversive suggestions not just because of the kind of thinking and doing they entail but also because of the chronotopes (or time rhetorics) they invoke. More simply, these classes don't clock onto quick progressions and performances, or timed accumulations of knowledge. They don't follow the rigid timetabling of Rothman's asylums.

On the other hand, in each of these movies the filmic device of the montage highlights speed and performance. In all of these movies, the montage is used to narrate overcoming, often against the analogue back-drop of the athletic contest (individual triumph at the expense of others, races, timed quizzes, or debates).[25] Both the athletic backdrop and the accelerated time of the montage say revealing things about the univer-sity, as the inverse of crip time and of accessible pedagogy, as a place that is both rigid and rushed in a manner that makes learning seem exceed-ingly stressful and difficult, if possible at all. As Dean Barbe says in *Back to School*, "there are two types of people in business today, the quick and the dead"—and this seems to apply to the university as well.

In general, crip time and the montage fall at two ends of the spectrum of filmic time. Filmic time can be understood as the temporal ordering and arrangement of events in film, to fit the action into 100 minutes— and this is generally quite different from "real time." It gets called "filmic time" because the people who think about film generally write about it in ways that makes film theory hard to understand. But also because time is a subjective thing. Time, something that we think of as needing to be uniform, standard, and normal, actually is subjective, experienced differently by different people, and malleable. Sound familiar? Yes, like the body itself, time can only cling to a fantasy of normality. So we need modifiers to properly understand time. There is no one type of time— instead, for example, there is academic time, and there is film time, the time constraints that films have to fit into, but also the version of time that film argues for.

One of the key ways we control and shape the experience of time is through mediums like long-form Hollywood films. So we need terms like "filmic time" because they show us that movies shape time in particular ways. They plot lives and relationships and communities and societies out in relatively short—100 minute—bursts. The ways that popular film plots out these bursts of time tends to be normative. So when I use the term "filmic time" I am also saying "normate time": the ways that time disciplines the experience of disability and the ways that disability can only appear in a prescriptive, limited when.

Generally, disabled characters are shown as a drag upon filmic time: too fast, too slow, always held in the "not-yet" space of disability, man-dated by its "not-me" status (Titchkosky "The Becoming"; Garland-

Thomson "Extraordinary"). So disabled characters usually either die or are cured when a film is sequenced in a normative way.

But even when there are flashbacks and flash-forwards and dream sequences, disabled characters often get depicted as obsessing about memories of their previously able selves or dreaming of cures and normative futures. One of the main ways that mainstream film controls and shapes perceptions of time is through its treatment of the disabled body. For decades, seeing a disabled character in almost any genre of film was like seeing a ticking time bomb—that character would need to be cured, or die, before the end of the film. Someone famously said that there are no second acts in American lives. Well, there have also generally been no second acts in the lives of disabled characters on-screen. When a disabled character is cured, they are cured because the viewer needs to believe that they themselves would be cured—or would compensate, or would overcome—if they became disabled. Perhaps even more disturbingly, when disabled characters die, there is the satisfaction of another kind of fantasy, perhaps eugenic. This extends so far as to affect the casting of films: every time a disability is depicted by a nondisabled actor, the audience is already jumping ahead to that actors' next able-bodied role, their disability drop. And Moore followed this script carefully in her Oscar acceptance speech.

Yet I want to end this chapter by suggesting that perhaps the ultimate fantasy of education in these films, and in popular culture, is that learning itself has a predictable narrative arc or sequential chronology, that it takes place across normate time, across campuses that we will always be at home in, or will always be recognizable to us—and that this narrative somehow makes us all more able (even slowly, through the gradual progression of "positive eugenics"). Instead of seeing education as a process of accumulation and realization, transfer, continuity, coherence, or progression, maybe it is a process of recursion, forgetting, simultaneity, regression, chaos. My hope is that we can refocus on the failures and refusals sometimes driving, sometimes ghosting, these films. This chapter itself is a montage, a supercut, a dream sequence, a series of flashbacks, and at a certain point this is how we all experience any film—or any learning. Further, because through these films we spend so much actual time with the underdogs, with those constructed as disabled or shown to be disabled by the pedagogies we witness in these films, we can ultimately resist the fantasy of segregation and perhaps reframe the who, the how, and the when of higher education.

While these films drastically misrepresent college life, in many ways, these movies about university also know and show more about universities than universities themselves do—unwittingly, perhaps, but to great effect. That is, universities and their stakeholders are not aware of themselves as exclusionary. Instead, they paint themselves as diverse, albeit with careful curation. Every rejection and failure in higher education can be carefully justified, quantified, and legally explained by the organization, while in the movies and in the lives of actual students, they feel arbitrary, frequent, and personal. Universities will not admit their role in rape culture, even when they establish small committees of the powerless to address "sexual violence"—and large committees of powerful lawyers to perform the calculus required to avoid lawsuits. The curriculum and the pedagogy of the college instructor is closely guarded by standards and elitism and intellectual freedom, even when this teaching can take away the freedom of students and leaves them feeling confused, stressed, and ignored. In the end, perhaps we should trust Hollywood more than we trust the public relations departments of universities.

The classroom is a rhetorical space, one that must be read carefully and critically, and one that can be reshaped. The classroom is also a public and a "protopublic" space. Its forms, routines, modes, power dynamics, empowerments, opportunities, exclusions, inclusions, disablements, accommodations, designs, failures, successes, limits, and possibilities extend into the public sphere. Classrooms reflect and shape larger cultural and social trends. Higher education is a social experiment, eugenic experiment, economic experiment—and an experiment with human subjects, not just abstract ideas. This is the case outside of North American and Europe as well, as movies such as *Twenty* (South Korea) and *Three Idiots* (India) could just as easily have been the subjects of analysis in this chapter.

A protopublic space, the university is also increasingly a retroprivate space. That is, private industry leaders and private industry values get imported into academia to try and clean it up, or to wrest power away from the self-governance of academics. And, more and more often, higher education is a political pawn, a place where the protopublic potential of the classroom is harnessed by governors, premiers, and other politicians who understand that they can utilize the university to make ideological arguments. So they imperil tenure, or they cancel programs that they see as teaching only "political correctness." They harness the doubtful, skeptical, critical attitude of the public toward the university, knowing that they can gain a certain group of voters by attacking the elitism of the university. In this way, the politicians follow the lead of movies about higher education.

Yet these films also harness the positive energy that comes from learning, and the positive energy that results when students begin taking control of their own learning, often in opposition to the traditional regimes of education.

These films show, finally, that if rhetoric is the circulation of discourse through the body, then spaces and institutions cannot be disconnected from the bodies within them, the bodies they selectively exclude, and the bodies that actively intervene to reshape them. These fictional worlds also cannot distract us from recognizing and making space for the real bodies, the real students in, currently kept out of, accommodated within, or actively reshaping the future of higher education.

Commencement

Donald Trump, in a Trump University advertisement:

"At Trump University, we teach success. That's what it's all about—success."

The final edits for this book were completed in the last few weeks of the Trump-Clinton presidential race of 2016. For much of this time it was energizing to be doing this work. It felt relevant and useful to be writing about ableism when there was a presidential candidate so overtly harnessing its rhetorical force, wrapping it in sexism and racism and xenophobia. I felt like I was writing toward an audience that, in the wake of the public repudiation of Trump, might be increasingly receptive to this book's arguments and messages. I have been writing to reveal racism, sexism, homophobia and transphobia, and (of course) ableism, arguing that it was all tangled and systemic and powerful and pervasive. But I took the comfortable (privileged) position that things were getting better, that the world was getting closer to something like awareness, or equity. I thought: progress is being made.

Then Donald Trump won.

In the week after Trump won, there were powerful protests against Trump on college campuses. Rudy Giuliani, a potential Trump cabinet minister, in an interview in the week following the election, reacting to these campus protests, called students "a bunch of spoiled crybabies," and faculty "left-wing loonies" (Jaschik).

There were also examples of extreme racism, sexual harassment, and ableism in public schools, colleges, and universities. Trump supporters in Texas called for vigilantes to "go arrest & torture those deviant university leaders spouting off all this <u>Diversity Garbage</u>" (Cardona, emphasis in the original). Another message on a flyer called diversity "a [expletive] theory" that "tries to convince us that **quality** no longer matters" (Cardona, emphasis in the original).

In this book, I've argued that universities lobby for change through the invention of specific types of student (and faculty) minds and bodies. So it is possible that the students and faculty who support the kind of inclusiveness and diversity I have been arguing for in these pages will be constructed as "loony," "spoiled," low quality, and much worse in the coming years, as Trump and others reshape education. As mentioned in my last chapter, the public doesn't seem to like university administrators or professors, and also seems to dislike the students for whom success at college or university seems natural and easy. In a climate in which academia is increasingly under fire for "coddling" students, for promoting identity politics, for being too "liberal," it will be increasingly important to better understand these critiques.

The world will have an American president who was elected despite his open mocking of disability, despite the fact that he was caught bragging on tape about sexual assault, despite the fact that he promised to deport Muslims and Mexicans, despite the fact that he has shown an allegiance to eugenic ideology (access D'Antonio), despite the fact that he ran a for-profit university himself that "the highest legal officer in New York State has described as a classic bait-and-switch scheme" (Cassidy).

Further, on February 7th of 2017, the U.S Senate confirmed Betsy DeVos as the 11th Secretary of Education. Quickly, DeVos moved to remove legislation aimed at holding for-profit colleges accountable for the federal funding they receive. Further, the department of education manages nearly $2 trillion in loans and grants, the largest student aid budget in its 37-year history. DeVos will be responsible for this huge economic portfolio. We know that disabled students are likely to have up to 60 percent more student debt by the time they graduate (Mohamed n.p.). If, as expected, DeVos removes the regulations and measures of accountability from that huge $2 trillion student aid portfolio, disabled students are likely to be disproportionately impacted—there will be less consequences attached to extending and elongating the path to degrees for these students, and at the same time there will be incentives attached to these elongations for lenders and educational institutions—both of whom stand to benefit financially. Thus the ways that disabled students are "marked out for wearing out" in higher education will also become the same means for lenders and for schools to profit. The managerial class on college campuses promises to expand in a world in which access to financial aid and loans is likely to become unfettered—you'll need more executives to maximize the exploitation of these programs. It is certain that the drop in scholarship money and the general increase in student debt impacts disabled students disproportionately.

Especially chilling is that fact that DeVos and her family have clear financial ties to Performant Financial Group, a company specializing in buying bad student loans (access Douglas-Gabriel). Performant and companies like it are the vultures circling higher education.

We can also assume that the historical articulation of federal rights and protections for disabled people in education will be hurt by the appointment of Betsy DeVos. During her confirmation hearing, DeVos seemed to have little or no knowledge at all of the IDEA, The Individuals with Disabilities Education Act (IDEA)—a four-part piece of American legislation that ensures students with a disability are provided with Free Appropriate Public Education that is tailored to their individual needs. In a letter, following this dismal showing on the Senate Floor, DeVos clarified that she wants to provide students with disabilities more educational opportunities. As she has done over and over again in other moments, she praised a voucher program, this time one that helps K-12 students with disabilities attend private school funded with taxpayer dollars: "One additional strategy I will pursue is to look for ways to increase access by students with disabilities to a broader range of educational options. I have seen exciting changes in students with disabilities when they attend schools that meet their needs" (qtd. in Strauss). She then went on to discuss the case of a family friend in great detail, and praised the Jon Peterson Special Needs Scholarship program in Ohio, which gives public funds to eligible K-12 students who have IEPs (individualized education plans, crucial to access at the K-12 level) to attend the private school of their choice. That program, as well as many other voucher programs, require participating families to agree to give up special education due-process rights they are given under the IDEA law. In this way, in a letter designed to prove to Senators and the public that she understood and would defend the IDEA, she was in fact advocating for programs in which students forego these hard-fought rights (Strauss).

Currently introduced on the house floor (as of March 2017), HR 610 or the "Choices in Education Act of 2017," proposes to fund (through block grants) elementary and secondary education only if states "comply with education voucher program requirements." And, as the National Council on Disability has shown, "IDEA rights, as a general rule, [do] not extend to children and youth with disabilities who participate in voucher programs. Section 504 of the Rehabilitation Act and the Americans with Disabilities Act will still apply to the administration of the voucher program but not to most activities of the private school" (Sailor and Stowe, 1). It is altogether possible that such waiving of rights could occur at the college and university level in the future. But the impact is also rhetorical: the idea is that segregation is best.

We already know that, in the U.S, some studies show that two-thirds of college students "don't receive accommodations simply because their colleges don't know about their disabilities" (Grasgreen n.p.). Those who do seek accommodations are likely to do so only in their third or fourth year of school. So, whatever the statistics tell us about how dire prospects might be for disabled students, the statistics only speak for the very small number of disabled students who successfully navigate the complicated accommodation process to seek help. When you introduce the idea that the best way for students with disabilities to learn is not to change their schools to become more accommodating and less ableist, but instead for students to "attend schools that meet their needs," then we enter dangerous terrain. So far, in higher education, the inclusion of disabled students in regular classrooms, when they are included at all, has been the norm. But the U.S now has an education secretary who has only ever publicly commented on disabled students when championing segregated schools and segregated programs. We should—very unfortunately—expect these schools and programs to thrive.

Academic Ableism, indeed.

In the face of very overt and popular ableist attacks on and reshapings of higher education, I worry that allegiance to a respectable and polite form of ableist rhetoric will also be much easier. Faculty and students may continue to be rewarded for ableist apologia, for defending ableism, and thus capable of protecting the privilege of the university themselves, and retaining their positions. There will also be many reasons not to protest, not to argue for greater diversity, not to protect or organize with vulnerable students or colleagues, not to risk your own disclosures. Students and teachers will likely continue to show allegiance to the exclusions that reinforce their privilege, and show allegiance to processes that maintain that privilege. Disability on campus may thus continue to exist only as a negative, private, individual failure. The university may never be a space held responsible for causing disability. Disability may instead continue to be seen to exist prior to, to remain external to, and to be remedied or erased according to only the arm's-length accommodations of a blameless and secure academic institution.

Clearly, there is a lot of work to do.

So what can I do? What can you do, if you care about creating a more inclusive, less discriminatory academy, one that refuses the eugenic legacy of higher education?

First, if you are about to teach, access the appendix to this book that is available on the University of Michigan Press site (www.press.umich.edu), and choose a Universal Design teaching idea and bring it into your classroom. Also, try to follow the principles of Universal Design for diversity discussed in this book.

If you are a faculty member or an administrator who might be in the powerful position of considering or supporting the disability accommodations of a colleague, or if you are ready to ask for the accommodations that you will almost undoubtedly need at some point in your career, read Margaret Price's "It Shouldn't Be So Hard" [https://www.insidehighered.com/advice/2011/02/07/margaret_price_on_the_search_process_for_those_with_mental_disabilities] and read Stephanie L. Kerschbaum et al., "Faculty Members, Accommodation, and Access in Higher Education" [https://profession.mla.hcommons.org/2013/12/09/faculty-members-accommodation-and-access-in-higher-education/], published in *Profession* in 2013. In the open access version of this book, these links will be provided.

When your university launches their mental health awareness day or week, or gives you a shirt or a button or a sticker to wear for wellness, use social media, the classroom, and other venues to also question what the structural issues are on your campus that actually need attention and funding because they might even cause exclusion—rather than downloading the demand for wellness and health onto individuals.

If there are laws like the ADA or AODA governing your campus, call attention to noncompliance.

If you are about to publish something, read Carl Straumsheim's article on guidelines for publishing accessible books, [https://www.insidehighered.com/news/2015/11/03/u-michigan-press-endorses-accessible-book-book-publishing-guidelines].

If you might be involved in hiring, read this article on creating accessible hiring practices: "Wanted: Disabled Faculty Members," [https://www.insidehighered.com/advice/2016/10/31/advice-hiring-faculty-members-disabilities-essay], published in *Inside Higher Education* in 2016.

If you are working on a syllabus, look at these examples that can help you move beyond simply retrofitting a disability "statement" onto this document:

Tara Wood and Shannon Madden, "Suggested Practices for Syllabus Accessibility Statements," *Kairos: A Journal of Rhetoric, Technology, and Pedagogy* [http://kairos.technorhetoric.net/praxis/tiki-index.php?page=Suggested_Practices_for_Syllabus_Accessibility_Statements]. Or spend some time on the Accessible Syllabus Project [https://accessiblesyllabus.tulane.edu/] website.

If you coordinate or administer a program, or otherwise are ready to begin to sync up your curriculum with disability accommodations that aren't just defeat devices, access this example letter designed to help you work with the office of disability services on your campus to expand accommodations and ensure that they are actually appropriate to your teaching:

Tara Wood, Melissa Helquist, and Jay Dolmage, "Accommodation Addenda: Expanding Possibilities for Inclusion." (www.URL TO COME)

If you are planning a conference or preparing to share your work at a conference, visit the Composing Access project [https://u.osu.edu/composingaccess/] to learn how you can make your conference and your conference presentation more accessible.

The steep steps of higher education will not easily be torn down or ramped over. The eugenic legacies that schools are built upon won't easily be refuted and are more likely to be strongly reinforced in the coming years. The structural inequities in place before students even make their way to the approaches and the gates will be actively ignored or more deeply entrenched. But no matter what you are about to do, there are real resources to help you avoid the ableism inherent in doing so. No matter what you are about to do, the work ahead is bound to be difficult. In fact, as teachers and students we know our failures are guaranteed; but we also know they can be powerfully rhetorical, powerfully meaningful.

There will always be disabled students in your class, and disabled faculty on your campus. Such a student or faculty member may already—or in the future—be you. We must imagine a future in which disability does not need to be denied or hidden or tokenized or erased.

Universities construct themselves (or Hollywood constructs them) as perhaps the most rigid and traditional of social structures. Others want to construct universities and professors as, inversely, radical, full of special snowflakes and political partisans. The only certainty is that how teaching and curriculum are built will also shape a broader geography, a wider public, and will always be subject to design and redesign.

For reasons of space, and by choice, and because of the speed of change, this book has certainly failed to cover many relevant topics, and has certainly failed to do many, many things. But hopefully it hasn't failed to give you ways to change higher education, starting today.

Notes

—— ⚓ ——

Introduction

1. Throughout the book when I mention another source that the reader might find interesting, instead of writing "see Hunter" I will use the term "access." Throughout the book I will also, more generally, make an effort to avoid relying on metaphors of sight or hearing.

2. The recent successful push from students and faculty to have Columbia University divest from private prisons is a story with a good ending, yet it underscores the fact that this is one of the only universities to do so; many others are heavily invested.

3. Take, for example, the recent story of Jasmin Simpson, a student who exposed the ways that the Canada Student Loans Program discriminates against students with disabilities.

4. This data is, admittedly, old—but there are reasons to believe that the situation is actually currently worse than it was 8–10 years ago. We also should ask why it is so difficult to access this type of data. Educators are engaged hyperactively in quantifying the benefits of higher education but very little data can be found on its failures.

5. This extends to the culture around seeking help for mental health issues. As Daniel Eisenberg, Ezra Golberstein, and Sarah Gollust show, "even in an environment with universal access to free short-term psychotherapy and basic health services, most students with apparent mental disorders did not receive treatment" (594). Their study showed that "of students with positive screens for depression or anxiety, the proportion who did not receive any services ranged from 37% to 84%" (594).

6. There are a variety of ways to tackle this clear discrimination against disabled faculty. One way is to overhaul academic hiring practices. Access, for instance, the article "Wanted: Disabled Faculty" by Stephanie Kerschbaum and myself in *Inside Higher Education*. Another key problem lies in the legalistic and minimalistic approach to accommodating faculty, a process that is perhaps even worse than the process for accommodating students. Access "Faculty Members, Accommodation, and Access in Higher Education," an article cowritten by Kerschbaum, myself, and many others and published in *Profession* in 2013 (Oswal et al.)

7. Organisation for Economic Co-Operation and Development (OECD) data shows that in 2009, "almost 3.7 million tertiary [higher education] students were enrolled outside their country of citizenship" (n.p.).

8. Later, when I write about the concept of Universal Design, I will discuss the concepts of "responsive design," in which we expect to be able to access content across devices; positive redundancy, in which it is valuable to have access to multiple iterations of content; and tolerance for error, in which good design allows us to use a technology or an object in a variety of ways without failing or simply giving up. Plain language, the way I am trying to implement it in this book, hopefully will accomplish a lot of these objectives as well. Plain language should allow readers a variety of ways of accessing ideas without being left behind or left out.

9. Consider, for instance, what you have to do to get an accessible format of an article for a student, if that article were published in a Routledge or Taylor & Francis non-Open-Access, expensive, very proprietary journal. You have to join a disturbingly euphemistic club called "Academic VIPs," disclose that student's name and the fact that they have a "visual (or physical) impairment, or a learning difficulty" (access Taylor and Francis, n.p.). There are then a long series of legal provisions and rules. There doesn't appear to be any provision at all for a faculty member with a disability seeking accessible formats; though it can be assumed that these teachers would also be compelled to disclose their disability. Not only is access not "open" in such a scheme, but the disabled person is forced to disclose that disability, or the teacher is forced to extend access as an act of charity or stewardship. The human "right to know" is significantly impeded (Willinsky, 7).

10. In Canada, it wasn't much better: only 57 percent of pages used text equivalents, 55 percent followed basic HTML guidelines, and only 25 percent of pages "passed" basic navigational tests (Thompson et al.).

Chapter 1

1. Access Peter Jacobs; more on this in the final chapter.

2. Hudson is the cofounder of Black Lives Matter Toronto and former executive director of University of Toronto Students' Union.

3. As Astra Taylor points out, "over 100 billion dollars of educational endowment money nationwide is invested in hedge funds, costing [schools] approximately $2.5 billion in fees in 2015 alone. The problems with hedge funds managing college endowments are manifold, going well beyond the exorbitant—some would say extortionate—fees they charge for their services" and include "the problem of conflict of interest on endowment boards of both public and private colleges" (n.p.). Some Ivy League schools end up paying hedge fund managers two to three times as much as they spend on tuition assistance and fellowships (Taylor, n.p.). Sometimes, these hedge fund managers are also members of their boards of trustees (Taylor, n.p.).

4. If such offices truly cared about wellness, they might work to make healthy food more available on campuses, and subsidize it. A recent study found that 39 percent of Canadian students experience food insecurity, with "Aboriginal and racialized peoples, off campus dwellers, and students that primarily fund their education through government student financial assistance programs experience[ing] exceptionally high rates of food insecurity" (Silverthorn, n.p.). An American study found that food-insecure students reported lower GPAs (Maroto, Snelling, and Linck, n.p.). Single parents, African American or multiracial students experienced the greatest

food insecurity (Maroto, Snelling, and Linck, n.p.). Unsurprisingly, food insecurity led to lower energy and concentration (Maroto). Food insecurity also led to higher rates of depression, disordered eating, and suicidal thoughts (Goldrick-Rab, Broton, and Eisenberg).

5. ADAPT is an activist organization that started as American Disabled for Accessible Public Transit, www.adapt.org. Following successful protests for the right to public transportation, and following a perceived shift toward greater access, the group has come to focus on the right to personal support services, and has renamed itself American Disabled for Attendant Programs Today, "fighting so people with disabilities can live in the community with real supports instead of being locked away in nursing homes."

6. This protest was memorialized and repeated by ADAPT in April 2009.

7. So-called postmodern disability studies contradicts this British philosophy by suggesting that the strict separation of impairment and disability is an illusion or a lie. The social model suggests the existence of both physical impairment and cultural disablement as engaged, yet independently sovereign or separate, truths. The postmodern model blurs the lines between the two. This philosophy interrogates the ways that bodies and cultures, biology and social structures—even texts—interact and cocreate one another. Much as Judith Butler has troubled the natural/cultural binary of sex and gander, this postmodern model has troubled the notion of natural bodies; the very idea of a body separate from culture. Judith Butler's definition of a "partial" social construction of the body, from her introduction to *Bodies That Matter*, nicely distills this idea: "to claim that discourse is formative is not to claim that it originates, causes, or exhaustively composes that which is concedes; rather, it is to claim that there is no reference to a pure body which is not at the same time a further formation of that body" (5). Any reference to a body is also a formation of that body. In this way, every formation is a further metaphor—these metaphors, in referencing the "pure body," may fortify it, while new metaphors might reform it.

8. Though Canada has no real equivalent to the ADA, smaller acts like the Accessibility for Ontarians with Disabilities Act (AODA) are already being framed in terms of legal minima and potential fines, not rights and responsibilities; and the backlash has been strong.

9. This repeats the historical pattern of disability and the experience of being disabled being negatively shaped and delimited by those who hold the cultural capital that allows them to pose (at least temporarily) as able-bodied. It is possible, then, that the university/institution binary simply gets reproduced within the university itself. The reality is that one cannot truly be included in any world until their input also shapes that world. As Brendan Gleeson has written, "disabled people in Western societies have been oppressed by the production of space . . . due in part to their exclusion from the discourses and practices that shape the physical layout of societies" (2). Or, as Sharon Snyder and David Mitchell write, "we cannot know a culture until we ask its disabled citizens to assess it" (Narrative, 178).

10. For instance, the term "moron" was invented by Henry Goddard in 1910, and the classification was key to research he performed on immigrants at Ellis Island beginning in 1913. As Anna Stubblefield has argued, Goddard's invention of this term as a "signifier of tainted whiteness" was the "most important contribution to the concept of feeble-mindedness as a signifier of a racial taint," through the diagnosis of the menace of alien races, but also as a way to divide out the impure elements of the white race (173, 162).

Chapter 2

1. As a result, public understanding of the ADA casts those who seek the protection of the law along the lines of, as Johnson notes, "the alligator in the sewers of New York City, like the worms in the Big Mac" (132). Thus, in Johnson's words, "The ADA, despite the Supreme Court's actions, still has a core premise that has yet to be understood by society: that people called 'disabled' are just people—not critically different from the rest of us. In order to address disability discrimination the right way as a nation, we first have to come to grips with the underlying realities of human abilities and disabilities. . . . The goal is not to fixate on, overreact to or engage in stereotypes about such differences, but to take them into account and allow for reasonable accommodation for individual abilities and impairments that will permit equal participation" (150).

2. Later in the book, I will examine Lauren Berlant's concept of slow death to define this timing or chronicity. Slow death through "accommodation" and the supplemental logic of the retrofit would not be a way of "defining a group of individuals merely afflicted with the same ailment, [but rather] slow death describes populations marked out for wearing out" (Berlant, 760). Annika Konrad's term for this process is "access fatigue": "being plain sick of having to ask for access" (n.p.). Berlant uses the term "death" intentionally, and Konrad uses the term "sick" intentionally. The process of looking for access is itself, in a way, disabling.

3. More on the power imbalance of this type of student-teacher exchange (this circulation of power through bodies) later in the book.

4. Ireland, Dale. Personal Correspondence with the Author. 16 April 2016.

5. Selber, Stuart. Personal Correspondence with the Author. 10 February 2016.

6. If you are interested in using these texts as more than just retrofits, access Tara Wood and Shannon Madden's excellent *Kairos* piece on suggested best practices for these syllabus accommodation statements.

7. We could spend a long time talking about the trends in naming these offices and their uses of euphemisms and what Simi Linton called "nice words." I could also comment on the increasing overlap between these offices and other (often much better-funded) student "wellness" and "success" offices, both of which are exnominative. That is, the terms "student wellness" and "student success" name or demand their inverse: don't get ill or unwell; don't fail out and stop paying tuition.

8. I am writing mainly about students here. It is beyond the scope of this book—in a way—to fully discuss the ways that universities and colleges shape and react to disabled faculty and staff (or even, really, graduate students). I would hope that readers will be able to use some of what I offer in this book to begin to better understand these other roles and positions as well—because they are inseparable. Margaret Price and Stephanie Kerschbaum's ongoing *Disability Disclosure* project, examining the ways that college and university instructors disclose their disabilities, will surely break new ground in this area. Also of interest might be the coauthored "Faculty Members, Accommodation, and Access in Higher Education" published in *Profession* in 2013 (Oswal et al.).

9. As Michael Hiltzik wrote of the American disability benefits program in the *Los Angeles Times*, "perhaps because it covers a relatively small number of Social Security recipients, the disability program has always been a prime victim of mythmakers. Its beneficiaries are portrayed as slackers gaming the system like the Coen brothers' Jeff Lebowski, whiling away his life at the bowling alley and snarfing down White Russians" (n.p.). He goes on to contextualize: "these are all varieties of a fictional genre known as 'the undeserving poor' that encompasses Ronald Reagan's folksy

yarns about welfare queens living on six-figure welfare handouts. The goal is to ratio-nalize cuts in benefits by portraying their beneficiaries as morally depraved" (n.p.). There are similar logics on college campuses, as well as in the general public about what happens on college campuses.

Chapter 3

1. And as Harvey Graff points out, "'many literacies' sits precariously between an essential, and a necessary recognition, and the dangers of trivialization and debase-ment of literacy. Overuse of the term 'literacy' and the concepts empties it of value and useful meanings" (22).

2. Similarly, Kress and Leeuwen take the "multi-skilled person" capable of freely choosing between modes of expression as a given, a "point of departure" in order to move along to a study of multimodal semiotics (Multimodal Discourse, 2). It is also important to note that Selber is not uncritically invoking this ideal student. His entire book is written along the faults of the digital divide, and is centrally about how "teach-ers and students should be mindful of ways in which they can unwittingly promote inequitable and counterproductive technological practices" (8).

3. The Super student is who all universities want to showcase, want to build their image around: look at any modern university website, and shuffled among the faculty profiles and event announcements are profiles of these Super students. Their varied skills and achievements stand in for the goals of entire institutions.

4. As the New London Group writes: "the new fast capitalist literature stresses adaptation to constant change through thinking and speaking for oneself; critique and empowerment; innovation and creativity; technical and systems thinking; and learning how to learn . . . as new systems of mind control or exploitation" (Cope and Kalantzis, 12). These "market-directed theories and practices, though they may sound humane, will never authentically include a vision of meaningful success for all students" (Cope and Kalantzis, 12).

5. There is further magical thinking surrounding Super Samantha: the fantasy that these students can basically teach themselves, or even teach one another, or teach us.

6. At least we would hope not—though, of course, the defunding of public edu-cation, often something voted upon, tells a different story.

7. Access World Bank: "Government expenditure on education, total (% of GDP)."

8. The retrofit is also a logic of fast capitalism—fast capitalism is the tendency of capitalism to extract surplus value with as little investment as necessary for the great-est return, while adding as little to the real economy as possible, often by means of financial speculation and the quickening of production. Yet what gets produced gets less and less tangible, harder to measure. This fast capitalism is seen by some as the necessary consequence of capitalism—it keeps speeding up, keeps extracting value, keeps becoming more efficient, and continues to exact more and more affective and embodied—and environmental—costs. Like fast capitalism, the retrofit marketizes philanthropy and charity—the industry of temporarily correcting or normalizing dis-ability is massive, one of the largest and fastest growing industries in our modern world, encompassing global pharmaceutical and biotechnology corporations, as well as architects and lawyers and even educational "specialists." Like fast capitalism, the retrofit offers only a quick and temporary fix to critical sociopolitical and economic conditions, and it does so with a fix that offers next to nothing of practical use.

9. Their landmark edited collection *Disability Incarcerated*, among other things,

"shows that experiences of disabled people, and processes of disablement, are central to understanding the rationales, practices and consequences of incarceration" (Ben-Moshe, Chapman, and Carey, x). I would add that we cannot disconnect these rationales, practices, and consequences from higher education, as counterintuitive as that may at first seem.

10. Robert Davis and Mark Shadle, interestingly, also cast this as an existing and ongoing equity issue: "The most successful students are often those who cut across the grain to mix discourses in intelligent ways, despite the structure of the course, while those who struggle cannot find voices despite, or because of, being told how they should sound" (31). In this scheme, if we don't explicitly teach and assess multimodality and multiliteracy, we will just continue to tacitly penalize those who can't do it. Access also Hitt.

11. I have written elsewhere about how this metaphor of "slow thought" conditions cultural perceptions of disability by utilizing pseudoscientific premises about how the brain works (access Dolmage "Between the Valley and the Field").

12. Here I am borrowing from the idea of "racecraft": Barbara Fields and Karen Fields' coinage used to define how discussions of racism turn into discussions of race, how a conversation about poverty actually becomes a way to denigrate racial groups, how people can say racist things and still defend themselves by saying they weren't talking about race at all. So when former Canadian prime minister Stephen Harper praised "old stock Canadians," it appeared to many that he was actually denigrating newer groups of immigrants from non-Western countries. But he was able to defend himself and in fact label his critics as the racists.

13. As I have explored in other work, one of the pseudoscientific legacies of eugenics is that we now ally disability with "slowness." One particularly damaging metaphor is the word "retarded," which, when we examine it, suggests that some people think more slowly than others, as though anyone has ever timed the speed of thoughts moving through the brain; or as though some people are arrested in their development. Despite this, the word "retarded" has long been given a reified and unquestioned status as a scientific term. But any time a student is constructed as slow, this eugenic legacy is invoked and utilized (access Dolmage, Disability Rhetoric).

14. While an argument that more senses equals more learning could be used to impose unwarranted assessments of ability upon learners, there is little proof—and little to be gained from arguing—that one organization or utilization of these pathways is better than another, or that learning happens best when they are all "maxed out." This said, Gunther Kress also argues that, because a culture selects and privileges certain forms of embodied engagement, some will be "affectively and cognitively at an advantage over those whose preferred sensory modes are not valued or are suppressed in their culture" ("Multimodality," 187). Kress sees how this cultural exclusion works, and wouldn't fail to recognize that there is a short jump from this attribution of cultural exclusion—a disadvantage only when the social practice disadvantages—to the attribution of a cognitive, even a biological deficiency. I would argue that this may lead us to attribute disabilities to learners who don't have access to whatever comes to be defined as the full range of connected modes. So we must remain critical not just of which literacies a culture privileges, but also which combinations of literacies and which interactions between literacies come to represent advanced (or deficient) cognition

15. Sometimes, this comes down to the difference between process and product: if we remain amazed with the diverse multimodal products that great students can create, we neglect real inquiry into the multimodal processes of composing, regardless of output.

Chapter 4

1. Hopefully, there will soon be an archive of Mace's papers at North Carolina State, and thus an even more robust history of the Universal Design movement. Scholars such as Aimi Hamraie are at work on this history.

2. As I mentioned in my introduction, my hope is that the plain language approach to writing this book also creates things like tolerance for error, intuitive and flexible use, and so on.

3. We also know, based on my earlier discussion of "sick buildings," that the ability to carefully control climate in academic and other workplace buildings is part of what led to this sickness.

4. This tolerance for error also links to the "art of failure" that I will discuss in my final chapter.

5. If the goal is to test spelling, then the autocorrect metaphor may not work. But if the learning goal is larger than just spelling correctly, why would we make spelling the first barrier to participation?

6. I don't pretend here, or anywhere in this book, to know what "better" thinking is or what it looks like. In fact, I am trying to avoid cognitive approaches to teaching and learning as much as possible. I am not even certain that "more" thinking is better. What I am gesturing toward is that a different approach to teaching that allows for a wide variety of ways to think—slowly, quickly, and so on—is most likely to allow a wide range of students to learn.

7. One interesting offshoot of this reorientation of design thinking is Julian Bleecker's advocacy for "design fiction," a means of using science fiction scenarios to develop design ideas and to create empathy for other worlds. As I have written elsewhere, in science fiction, we are often asked to associate disability with future dystopia (access Dolmage, Disability Rhetoric). This said, looking at the ways that disability is represented in the work of Philip K. Dick, or Margaret Atwood, for instance, we might find ways to design hypothetical technologies that, instead of fixing disability, address what is dystopian about the cultural (and technological) construction of disability in these worlds. Such an activity would be excellent in a Literature, Disability Studies, or Design classroom.

8. Hopefully, stating this fact doesn't diminish the important ongoing design work of disabled folks such as Joshua Miele, creator of tactile maps, crowd-sourced video description, and DIY (do it yourself) hardware prototyping programs for the blind, developed out of the Smith-Kettlewell Eye Research Institute in San Francisco.

9. ADAPT is an activist organization that started as American Disabled for Accessible Public Transit, www.adapt.org. Following successful protests for the right to public transportation, and following a perceived shift toward greater access, the group has come to focus on the right to personal support services, and has renamed itself American Disabled for Attendant Programs Today, organizing disability rights advocates to engage in direct action on a variety of issues including housing, education and healthcare, in order to ensure the rights of people with disabilities.

10. Aside from this one classroom anecdote, there have been huge developments in design thinking in the last decade. For example, with the popularity of "responsive design," people expect the right to access content and media on whatever device they use. Can this extend to whichever body they use? The range of ways we think of what we might call design-for continue to expand. But we also get significant changes in how we think of design-by. For instance, Sara Hendren and Caitrin Lynch's recent *Engineering at Home* project shows that "an expanded view of engineering takes on new urgency . . . when it comes to design for disability. . . . Placing people at the center of

the research and development of 'assistive technologies' is critical to robust, innovative, adaptive engineering. Their project seeks to tell stories and provide examples of not just user-centered design but also 'user-initiated' design" (n.p). In their words, "perhaps especially in design for disability, attentive design-for-one practices can yield a powerful course correction to the top-down modes of manufacturing. A disposition of experimentation, a willingness to harvest the lessons of singularity, a provisional commitment to the one-off: these unique objects together form an argument for the recognition of more user-initiated technologies as engineering, wherever they originate and whatever market they may eventually find" (n.p.).

11. We then find very similar wording—a similarly affective description—of the feelings of people with disabilities who feel the International Symbol of Access (ISA)—the stick-figure wheelchair symbol—does not represent them. As Kelly Fritsch writes, "With the ISA, disability appears in order to disappear, is included to be excluded. The deployment of the ISA solves the problem of disability without ever needing to include disabled people or without ever needing to confront the contradictions of accessibility as it reduces 'the lived complexity' of disabled embodiment [into . . .] a thing that is contained and known; a stick figure in a blue box. In being known, disability can be taken care of by building ramps or, more importantly, simply by posting the ISA. That disability is taken care of is a good feeling. In this good feeling, ableism and compulsory able-bodiedness are covered over by happy affects. It is only when someone gets upset that these happy affects are disrupted. In these moments disability becomes a problem again" (n.p.).

12. Beacon College is a similar college to Landmark, aimed directly at students with learning disabilities. Their tuition is $31,916 a year, but they try to soften the blow by foregrounding the medical tax deductions families might get, just as other schools market federal student aid programs. Other programs like "Achieve," an online-only BA in liberal studies with an emphasis in computer science program at Sage College, are also marketed solely to students diagnosed with autism spectrum disorders. The tuition in the Achieve program starts at $27,000 for the first year, then a small jump in the second year, then to $43,000 in the third year, and another increase in the fourth year. Again, that's an astronomical cost for an online-only BA. The University of the Ozarks also offers special services for learning disabled students, at a cost of $22,900 a year, on top of the usual $23,750 tuition. Unsurprisingly, they actively recruit into the program (Krupnick, n.p.). It is also important to remember that it often costs around $5,000 to even get the testing done to verify a learning disability.

13. Neil Fitzgerald also writes about the similar "Passport" program at the University of Wisconsin. These geographic, immigration-tinged metaphors seem to be a trend in disability services offices, as the process of presenting accommodation letters over and over again is in many ways like "showing your papers."

14. Access Kimber Barber-Fendley and Chris Hamel's apologia for this program in *CCC* a few years back and my discussion of this in the last chapter.

15. The discourse about learning styles precedes the conversation around multiliteracy and multimodality, even as they overlap. And a key difference is that while learning styles are fairly overtly labeled as innate or unchanging, a matter of student biology, something that allows us to label a student and thus teach toward a series of differences, multimodality has more frequently been discussed as a goal: a flexibility that needs to be encouraged. You can have only one learning style (supposedly), but there is a kind of demand to have multimodality.

16. Further, Ellen Samuels shows how, within the "fantasies of identification" by which we try to classify bodies, disability is always "lurking at the margins of [these discourses] ready to be invoked to justify a range of oppressive and reductive identifica-

tions" (214). There are crises when we cannot easily and readily classify difference—and we react with fantasies that we can carefully identify things like sex and race and disability. But we also do this with different parts of the brain or with different types of brains—for instance, pop science seems obsessed with "the teen brain" (access Julie Elman's book Chronic Youth). According to Samuels, fantasies of identification "retroactively naturalize [their] determinative effects" (22). Such identifications search for "scientific underpinnings [and] homes" (214). More simply, we classify things first, and then we give them justifications that make the classification look scientific.

17. Ireland, Dale. Personal Correspondence with the Author. 16 April 2016.

Chapter 5

1. As Patrick Kinkade and Michael Katovich argue, "cult films are secular documents, celebrated as sacred texts by audiences and used as shared foci to collectively create rituals and belief systems. They differ from popular re-releases, fad films, films with cult qualities, and critical cult films in that they involve typical people in atypical situations, sympathetic deviance, challenges to traditional authority, reflections of societal strains, and paradoxical and interpretable resolutions" (n.p.).

2. As Jacinda Read shows, this sort of psychotronic reaction protects "laddish political incorrectness" and "legitimizes its anti-feminist and feminine tendencies through the reproduction, rather than analysis, of oppositional subcultural ideologies" (67). In short, saying that we need to ignore what's offensive in these films—because we all know they are offensive—and just focus on what's good about them is a way of actually legitimating their offenses.

3. There are ways that this segregation might provide opportunity for what Judith Halberstam and others call queer kinship: "relations that grow along parallel lines rather than upward and onward. This queer form of antidevelopment requires healthy doses of forgetting and disavowal and proceeds by way of a series of substitutions" (73). Yet the nerds most often are seen to reject the "Mus," and in most of these movies the possibility of queer kinship is pretty vexed. For instance, in Old School and Accepted, the protagonist "gets" the popular girl; the only overtly queer character is a caricature in Revenge of the Nerds; and yet an argument probably needs to be made about the intense homosociality of all of these films and how that interacts with the disability "closet" I mention in another part of this chapter.

4. Throughout this final chapter, instead of including movie stills and adding visual descriptions as "retrofits," I am going to omit the stills altogether, and instead only offer thick description.

5. As Jennifer Doyle argues, the phrase "rape culture" can be useful to "name places where sexual violence is explicit, frequent, rewarded" but "it can also distance us from the force of the ordinary" and the ongoing culture of sexual coercion on campuses (63).

6. As Doyle points out, this is tacit because "fraternity members [and other men] do not know how to narrate the centrality of sexual-coercion-by-men to their formation as men, or what it means to affirm that non-consensual sex forms the bedrock of their masculinity. They do not know how to reconcile their hatred of women with their certainty that they are not gay. They know even less what it means to resist the architecture of this entire scenario" (75).

7. We perceive this segregation, often, morphing into a form of elitism. This happens through the Harry Potter books and films, for instance, where there are clear differences between those who can go to Hogwarts and those who cannot, as well as between the different houses, leading to insufferable articles such as "If Hogwarts'

Houses Were Ivy League Schools." Further, as Michael Bérubé notes, there is a very important plot point that revolves around the disabled Ariana Dumbledore and her exclusion from school and social life (36). We could also discuss the Xavier Institute for Higher Learning in the *X-Men* films in a similar manner. I am isolating mention of Potter and X-Men to this footnote so as not to open up an entirely different can of worms, as fun as that might be.

8. I am very hesitant to retroactively diagnose Jordan here. My goal is not to do so in a way that newly stigmatizes her, or to suggest that we can't understand the character without the diagnosis. My goal in making this connection, however, is just to clearly show that the film codes all outsider characters with some form of embodied difference.

9. Lazlo is a "ticking time bomb" character in *Real Genius*, but he is also the one who figures out what the military uses of the laser that the students develop will be. He actually lives in a closet. There is a lot going on in *Real Genius* about the disability counterculture or shadow culture of the university, and the epistemology of the closet.

10. Perhaps the most arresting of these contrasts can be found in *With Honors*: Monty is a student, and when his computer crashes, he's left with only a single paper copy of his thesis, a thesis he needs to submit to graduate. Frightened of losing it, he immediately rushes out to photocopy it, only to stumble and drop it down a grate. Searching the basement of the building, he discovers that it has been found by Simon, a squatter. Simon makes a deal with Monty: for every day's accommodation and food that Monty gives him, he will give a page of the thesis in return.

11. *Revenge of the Nerds* comments on this in showing that the nerds become just as bad as the jocks after they have won—not "just the nerds they say we are," but also just like the jocks they said they hated. The underdogs, in these films, when these films have sequels, often become overdogs.

12. As Mary Nguyen showed in a 2012 study on how students balance debt, they are often involved in a "complex calculation, and students may not always make the best choices. Some students may borrow the entire cost of college, including living expenses, as a means of successfully earning a degree, only to default on loans that are too large to repay. Other students might not borrow enough money, taking on so much remunerative work that they don't devote enough time to their studies and end up dropping out. . . . risk factors among non-borrowers who dropped out were substantially higher than those among borrowers who dropped out, with almost three times as many non-borrowers enrolled part time their first year and then dropped out. The presence of these risk factors is often cited by colleges as an excuse for high student loan default rates, which are used by federal regulators to judge whether programs should be eligible for federal student aid. But it's important to note that these risk factors are not static traits. . . . they are behaviors, choices that students make, in significant part, in response to college prices. If colleges weren't so expensive, they wouldn't have as many working students with some combination of debt and work-related risk factors for dropping out" (n.p.).

13. Again, the monsters are mostly all men, and coded as white; the only major female character in the movie is the Dean Hardscrabble, who is dark purple and thus coded as African American. It is worth noting that her name—and her tough attitude—seem to denote the idea that she has worked very hard for the privilege she has been able to access, and has no patience for others who won't or can't work as hard.

14. In an earlier footnote, I discussed Julian Bleecker's concept of "design fiction": using sci-fi novels to help design students conceptualize a more diverse future

world. This entire chapter might be used in a similar way. How could *Monsters University*, for example, be used as design fiction: create a campus space and pedagogy that would actually work for these monsters.

15. The administrators, of course, are shown to be evil. Deans Barbe and Hardscrabble and the ones from *Old School, Accepted*, and *Animal House*, are all stuffy, traditional, and out to fail and expel. They talk about handpicking their students from the "crème de la crème" and they have absolute power and authority over everything from the size of the lawn to individual admissions decisions. They have lots of money and they are invested in maintaining their privilege. Dean Martin is shown to be a pushover, out for the money, but the other deans are also shown to be in someone's pocket—usually the Greek system or the football coach. Dean Barbe is the only dean who seems to also teach. Kieran Healy seems to agree, pointing out that "the role of Dean Hardscrabble in the everyday life of the university is particularly disturbing. She seems to feel it her right to observe and even interrupt lectures in progress, to overrule the teaching decisions of tenured faculty monsters, and to generally interfere with the curriculum's content and standards whenever she feels like it. It is a generally accepted rule of university governance that the faculty control the curriculum, and yet here we can recognize administrative interference on a very worrying scale. She also is clearly far too involved in the extracurricular life of the school, and in particular with its powerful fraternity and sorority culture. Moreover, the fact that there is a statue to Dean Hardscrabble placed inside the main lecture theater of the school which she administers bespeaks of a level of administrative hubris rarely seen outside of certain English universities. It is difficult to see how the faculty could be expected to work under such a dysfunctional managerial style" (n.p.).

16. Healy continues: "One has to wonder whether Monsters University recruits these talented young giant monsters for anything other than their athletic ability" (n.p). There is much more to be said about this, of course. Every one of these movies places sports, particularly football, at the very center of campus culture, and although most of the movies paint the athletes in a negative light, the pervasiveness and power of athletic culture on campus, hinged to fraternity culture, shows just how powerfully these institutions have stamped themselves on the public perception of college, to the exclusion of all other campus cultures.

17. This said, Downey's character is shown to be involved in protest, and he calls football a metaphor for nuclear war (and this was before Don DeLillo's *End Zone*). There is also a subgenre of Vietnam era films about college that look at protest culture, and perhaps Downey's character borrows from this genre. In fact, most of these movies steal from that genre but have their characters protesting for individual goals, not political ones.

18. Another place where this meritocracy is critiqued is through the application process: "I don't have a clue [what to do with the rest of my life]" is Bartleby's entrance essay in *Accepted*. The entire movie *Admission* is about the process, and how an officer in the admissions department at an Ivy League school is convinced to consider alternative forms of knowledge and success in students from underfunded schools. There is in fact a genre of admissions movies, films like *Orange County, Risky Business, The Spectacular Now, Me and Earl and the Dying Girl*. Each of these films focuses on the college admissions letter as a framing device and even as a narrative technique. Trying to figure out how to write a letter that will get them into college is a means of kick-starting self-reflection and development. Amy Vidali studies such letters for their normative power, and the films use the prospect of going to school or getting into school as means of making characters grow up, realize their true priorities, or focus on their dreams—they don't even need to set foot on campus to be conditioned by

204 · Notes to Pages 171–80

the selectivity and the norms of academia. Many of these movies are also about how these potential students might be able to even afford to go to college in the first place. In *Stealing Harvard*, the plot is driven by the need to deliver a girl from her lower station in life, and, as you might predict, theft becomes the only feasible solution.

19. In *Old School*, this takes the form of "The Charter Certification Review," given by the board of trustees: comprised of academics, athletics, community service, debate, and school spirit. In *Accepted*, there is a similar accreditation hearing in front of "state board of education." In *The House Bunny* and *Revenge of the Nerds* the accreditation board is made up entirely of Greek leaders.

20. The subversive nature of this move is undermined a bit or a lot by the fact that we know they will eventually bootstrap their way up in their new workplace, *Monsters Inc.*, as this is a prequel.

21. And they turn that into an actual class where all the men watch three women in bikinis float around in a pool; further literalizing the sexualized gaze that already exists in these films. As I mentioned before, women in these films don't seem to go to class, but they do go to parties.

22. This is accompanied by an antifaculty sentiment: "why don't you take your P-H-D and shove it up you're A-S-S" Dean Lewis yells at the dean of Harmon, and this sentiment can be tracked across all of these movies. Male professors are in general angry and incompetent or narcissistic and duplicitous and out to use their students (especially the misfits) for their own personal profit; female professors are, just like female students, sexual objects.

23. *Back to School* is also a statement of positionality: popular culture has its back to school. There is work to be done to argue that schools actually shape cultures, though without a doubt we can recognize the resistant attitude that the general public has towards school culture. Access, for instance, Andrew Ross's *No Respect: Intellectuals and Popular Culture*.

24. Jeffrey J. Williams goes so far as to argue that in these films "the university is generally not depicted as an ivory tower; it is a transformative zone toward full participation in adult life and in fact is often a public sphere in its own right. . . . University fiction, even in parody, takes the social position of the university seriously" (24).

25. Access *Rudy, He Got Game, Blue Chips,* and so forth. We should also note that *Rudy* is the *Rocky* of university films—he doesn't just overcome his stature to get onto the football field, he also overcomes dyslexia.

Bibliography

Accepted. Dir. Steve Pink. Universal, 2006.

Adjunct, Alice K. "The Revolving Ramp: Disability and the New Adjunct Economy." *Disability Studies Quarterly* 28.3 (2008).

Aguirre, Regina T. P., and Chad Duncan. "Being an Elbow: A Phenomenological Autoethnography of Faculty-Student Collaboration for Accommodations." *Journal of Teaching in Social Work* 33.4–5 (2013): 531–51.

Ahmed, Sara. "Feminist Killjoys (and Other Willful Subjects)." *Scholar and Feminist Online* (2010).

Ahmed, Sara. "Melancholic Universalism." *Feministkilljoys.com*, December 15, 2015; accessed March 7, 2016.

Ahmed, Sara. *On being included: Racism and diversity in institutional life.* Duke University Press, 2012.

Alexander, Michelle. *The New Jim Crow: Mass Incarceration in the Age of Colorblindness.* New York: New Press, 2012.

Allen, I. E., and J. Seaman. *Staying the Course: Online Education in the United States.* Needham, MA: Sloan Consortium, 2008.

American Association of University Professors. "Report on the Economic Status of the Profession." *Academe* 99.2 (March–April 2013).Aristotle. *Rhetoric.* Translated by J. H. Freese. Cambridge: Harvard University Press, 1926.

Aspen Institute. *Glossary for Understanding the Dismantling of Structural Racism.* Washington, DC: Aspen Institute, 2013.

Atleo, E. Richard. *Principles of Tsawalk: An Indigenous Approach to Global Crisis.* Vancouver, BC: UBC Press, 2012.

Aubrecht, Katie. "Psy-Times: The Psycho-Politics of Resilience in University Student Life." *Intersectionalities: A Global Journal of Social Work Analysis, Research, Polity, and Practice* 5.3 (2016): 186–200.

Back to School. Dir. Alan Metter. MGM, 1986.

Ball, Cheryl E. "Pirates of Metadata: The True Adventures of How One Journal Editor and Fifteen Undergraduate Publishing Majors Survived a Harrowing Metadata-Mining Project." In *Common Ground at the Nexus of Information Literacy and Scholarly*

Communication, edited by Stephanie Davis-Kahl and Merinda Kaye Hensley, 93–111. Chicago: Association of College and Research Libraries, 2013.

Banks, Joy. "Barriers and Supports to Postsecondary Transition Case Studies of African American Students with Disabilities." *Remedial and Special Education* 35.1 (2014): 28–39.

Baraka, Amiri. "Spike Lee at the Movies." *Black American Cinema*, edited by Manthia Diawara, 145–53. New York: Routledge, 1993.

Barber-Fendley, Kimber, and Chris Hamel. "A New Visibility: An Argument for Alternative Assistance Writing Programs for Students with Learning Disabilities." *College Composition and Communication* 55:3 (2004): 504–35.

Baynton, Douglas C. "Bringing Disability to the Center: Disability as an Indispensable Category of Historical Analysis." *Disability Studies Quarterly* 1 (Summer 1997): N.p. http://dsq-sds.org/article/view/108/108

Beckstead, Rachel. "College Dropout Statistics." *College Atlas*, August 14, 2014; accessed November 3, 2016.

Bell Jr, Derrick A. "Brown v. Board of Education and the Interest-Convergence Dilemma." *Harvard Law Review* (1980): 518–33.

Ben-Moshe, Liat, Chris Chapman, and Allison Carey, eds. *Disability Incarcerated: Imprisonment and Disability in the United States and Canada*. New York: Springer, 2014.

Berlant, Lauren. *Cruel Optimism*. Durham, NC: Duke University Press, 2011.

Berrett, Ann. "Manju Banerjee: Why I Moved to a College That Focuses on Students with Disabilities." *Chronicle of Higher Education*, April 1, 2012; accessed November 14, 2016.

Bérubé, Michael. *The Secret Life of Stories: From Don Quixote to Harry Potter, How Understanding Intellectual Disability Transforms the Way We Read*. NYU Press, 2016.

Bleecker, Julian, and Nicolas Nova. *A Synchronicity: Design Fictions for Asynchronous Urban Computing*. New York: Architectural League of New York, 2009.

Bolt, David. *Disability, Avoidance and the Academy: Challenging Resistance*. New York: Routledge, 2015.

Bousquet, Mark. *How The University Works*. New York: NYU Press, 2008.

Bowe, Frank G. *Universal Design in Education: Teaching Non-traditional Students*. Westport, CT: Bergin and Garvey, 2000.

Brand, Stewart. *How Buildings Learn: What Happens after They're Built*. London: Penguin, 1995.

Branson-Potts, Hayley. "UC Davis Chancellor Apologizes for Internet Scrubbing Controversy." *Los Angeles Times*, April 20, 2016; accessed November 1, 2016.

Brewer, Elizabeth, Melanie Yergeau, and Cynthia L. Selfe. "Creating a Culture of Access in Composition Studies." *Composition Studies* 42.2 (2014).

Brown, Lydia X. Z. "Ableism Is Not 'Bad Words.' It's Violence." *Autistic Hoya*, July 25, 2016; accessed November 1, 2016.

Brown, Wendy. *Undoing the Demos*. Brooklyn: Zone Books, 2015.

Brueggemann, Brenda Jo, and Georgina Kleege. "Gently Down the Stream: Reflections on Mainstreaming." *Rhetoric Review* 22.2 (2003): 174–84.

Brueggemann, Brenda Jo, Linda Feldmeier White, Patricia Dunn, Barbara A. Heifferon, and Johnson Cheu. "Becoming Visible: Lessons in Disability." *College Composition and Communication* (2001): 368–98.

Butler, Janine. "Where Access Meets Multimodality: The Case of ASL Music Videos." *Kairos: A Journal of Rhetoric, Technology, and Pedagogy* 22.1 (2016); accessed November 1, 2016.

Butler, Judith. *Bodies That Matter: On the Discursive Limits of Sex*. New York: Taylor and Francis, 2011.

Canguilhem, Georges. *Le normal et le pathologique*. Paris: Presses universitaires de France, 1966.

Cardona, Claire Z. "Texas State University Police Investigating Fliers Calling for 'Tar & Feather Vigilante Squads'." *Dallas News*, November 10, 2016; accessed November 12, 2016.

Carter, Angela M. "Teaching with Trauma: Trigger Warnings, Feminism, and Disability Pedagogy." *Disability Studies Quarterly* 35.2 (2015).

Casselman, Ben. "Race Gap Narrows in College Enrollment, but Not in Graduation." *FiveThirtyEight*, April 30, 2014; accessed April 9, 2016.

Cassidy, John. "Trump University: It's Worse Than You Think." *New Yorker*, June 2, 2016; accessed November 12, 2016.

Center for Excellence in Universal Design. "3 Case Studies on UD." January 1, 2012; accessed March 7, 2016.

Chapman, Chris, Allison C. Carey, and Liat Ben-Moshe. "Reconsidering confinement: interlocking locations and logics of incarceration." *Disability Incarcerated*. Palgrave Macmillan US, 2014. 3–24.

Chibnall, Steve. *Double Exposures: Observations on The Flesh and Blood Show*. In *Trash Aesthetics: Popular Culture and Its Audience*, edited by Deborah Cartmell, I. Q Hunter, Heidi Kaye, and Imedla Wheelan. London: Pluto Press, 1997.

Cogdell, Christina. *Eugenic Design: Streamlining America in the 1930s*. Philadelphia: University of Pennsylvania Press, 2010.

Cole, Emma & Stephanie Cawthon. "Self-Disclosure Decisions of University Students with Learning Disabilities." *Journal of Postsecondary Education and Disability*, 28.2 (2015): 163–79.

Cope, Bill, and Mary Kalantzis. *A Pedagogy of Multiliteracies*. London: Palgrave Macmillan UK, 2015.

Cortiella, Candace, and Sheldon H. Horowitz. "The State of Learning Disabilities: Facts, Trends, and Emerging Issues." New York: National Center for Learning Disabilities, 2014.

Cohen, Adam. *Imbeciles: The Supreme Court, American Eugenics, and the Sterilization of Carrie Buck*. Penguin Press HC, 2016.

Cowen, Tyler. "Autism as Academic Paradigm." *Chronicle of Higher Education*, February 13, 2009; accessed March 10, 2016.

Cushman, Ellen. "The Rhetorician as an Agent of Social Change." *College Composition and Communication* 47.1 (1996): 7–28.

D'Antonio, Michael. *The Truth about Trump*. New York: St. Martin's Griffin, 2016.

Daschuk, James William. *Clearing the Plains: Disease, Politics of starvation, and the Loss of Aboriginal life*. Regina, Sask.: University of Regina Press, 2013.

Davis, Lennard J. *Bending over Backwards: Essays on Disability and the Body*. New York: Verso, 1999.

Davis, Lennard J. *Enforcing Normalcy: Disability, Deafness, and the Body*. New York: Verso, 1995.

Davis, Robert L., and Mark F. Shadle. *Teaching Multiwriting: Researching and Composing with Multiple Genres, Media, Disciplines, and Cultures*. Carbondale: SIU Press, 2007.

Davis, Yumani. "The Normalization Process of Multimodal Composition: The 'Unseeing' People of Color." PhD diss., University of Central Florida, 2015.

Deleuze, Gilles. "Bartleby; or, the Formula." In *Essays Critical and Clinical*, translated by Daniel W. Smith and Michael A Greco, 68–90. Minneapolis: University of Minnesota Press, 1997.

Dewey, John. *Experience and Education*. New York: Collier Books, 1938.

Dolmage, Jay. "Between the Valley and the Field: Metaphor and 'Disability.'" *Prose Studies* 27.1 (Summer 2005): 108–19.

Dolmage, Jay. *Disability Rhetoric.* Syracuse: Syracuse University Press, 2014.

Dolmage, Jay. "Disability Studies Pedagogy, Usability and Universal Design." *Disability Studies Quarterly* 25.4 (2005).

Dolmage, Jay. "Disabled upon Arrival: The Rhetorical Construction of Race and Disability at Ellis Island." *Cultural Critique* 77 (Winter 2011): 24–69.

Dolmage, Jay. "Universal Design: Places to Start." *Disability Studies Quarterly* 35.2 (2015).

Dolmage, Jay, and Stephanie Kerschbaum. "Wanted: Disabled Faculty Members." *Inside Higher Education,* October 31, 2016; accessed November 14, 2016.

Douglas-Gabriel, Danielle. "Senator Wants to Help Homeless Students, Who Are 'Taking Out Loans for Survival'." *Washington Post,* November 12, 2015; accessed November 12, 2016.

Douglas-Gabriel, Danielle. "Dems raise concern about possible links between DeVos and student debt collection agency." *The Washington Post.* 17 Jan. 2017. Web. 24 Mar. 2017.

Doyle, Jennifer. *Campus Sex, Campus Security.* Boston: MIT Press, 2015.

Duffy, Elizabeth A., and Idana Goldberg. *Crafting a Class: College Admissions and Financial Aid, 1955–1994.* Princeton: Princeton University Press, 2014.

Duggan, Lisa. *The Twilight of Equality: Neoliberalism, Cultural Politics, and the Attack on Democracy.* Boston: Beacon, 2003.

Dunn, Patricia Ann. *Learning Re-Abled: The Learning Disability Controversy and Composition Studies.* Portsmouth, NH: Boynton/Cook, 1995.

Eisenberg, Daniel, Ezra Golberstein, and Sarah E. Gollust. "Help-Seeking and Access to Mental Health Care in a University Student Population." *Medical Care* 45.7 (2007): 594–601.

Ellis, Katie, and Gerard Goggin. "Disability, Locative Media, and Complex Ubiquity." In *Ubiquitous Computing, Complexity and Culture,* edited by Ulrik Ekman, Jay David Bolter, Lily Diaz, Morten Søndergaard, and Maria Engberg. New York: Routledge, 2015.

Elman, Julie Passanante. *Chronic Youth: Disability, Sexuality, and US Media Cultures of Rehabilitation.* New York: NYU Press, 2014

"Erasing Problem Does Not Equate to Fixing It." *The Daily Californian.* N.p., 07 Mar. 2017. Web. 10 Mar. 2017.

Erdur-Baker, Ozgur, John C. Barrow, Christopher L. Aberson, and Matthew R. Draper. "Nature and Severity of College Students' Psychological Concerns: A Comparison of Clinical and Nonclinical National Samples." *Professional Psychology: Research and Practice* 37.3 (2006): 317–23.

Erwin, Andrew, and Marjorie Wood. "The One Percent at State U: How Public University Presidents Profit from Rising Student Debt and Low-Wage Faculty Labor." Washington, DC: Institute for Policy Studies, 2014.

Fichten, Catherine S., Jennison V. Asuncion, Maria Barile, Chantal Robillard, Myrtis E. Fossey, and Daniel Lamb. "Canadian Postsecondary Students with Disabilities: Where Are They?" *Canadian Journal of Higher Education* 33.3 (2003): 71–130.

Fields, Barbara J., and Karen Fields. *Racecraft: The Soul of Inequality in American Life.* New York: Verso Books, 2012.

Findlay, Stephanie. "Whatever Happened to Tenure?" *Macleans.ca,* January 17, 2011; accessed March 2, 2016.

Fink, Shari, Steve Eder and Matthew Goldstein. "Betsy DeVos Invests in a Therapy Under Scrutiny." *The New York Times.* 30 Jan. 2017. Web. 27 Mar. 2017.

Fisher, Bonnie S., Leah E. Daigle, and Francis T. Cullen. *Unsafe in the Ivory Tower: The Sexual Victimization of College Women*. New York: Sage Publications, 2009.

Fitzgerald, F. Scott. *This Side of Paradise*. New York: Modern Library, 1996.

Fogg, Piper. "Grad-School Blues." *Chronicle of Higher Education* 55.24 (2009): B12–B16.

Ford, Star. "Deep Accessibility." *Ianology*, March 6, 2013; accessed March 10, 2016.

Foucault, Michel. *History of Sexuality I*. Translated by Alan M. Sheridan-Smith. New York: Pantheon, 1973.

Francavillo, Gwendolyn Suzanne Roberts. "Sexuality Education, Sexual Communication, Rape Myth Acceptance, and Sexual Assault Experience among Deaf and Hard of Hearing College Students." PhD diss., University of Maryland, 2009.

Freeman, Daniel. "Ableism and the Academy: What College Has Taught Me about My Disabled Body." *Model View Culture*, October 12, 2015; accessed March 10, 2016.

Freeman, Elizabeth. "*Monsters, Inc.*: Notes on the Neoliberal Arts Education." *New Literary History* 36.1 (2005): 83–95.

Fritsch, Kelly. "The Neoliberal Circulation of Affects: Happiness, Accessibility and the Capacitation of Disability as Wheelchair." *Health, Culture and Society* 5.1 (2013): 135.

Galton, Francis. *Essays in Eugenics*. 1985.

Garland-Thomson, Rosemarie. "The Case for Conserving Disability." *Journal of Bioethical Inquiry* 9.3 (2012): 339–55.

Garland-Thomson, Rosemarie. "Disability Studies: A Field Emerged." *American Quarterly* 65.4 (2013): 915–26.

Garland-Thomson, Rosemarie. *Extraordinary Bodies*. New York: Columbia University Press, 1996.

Garland-Thomson, Rosemarie. "Misfits: A Feminist Materialist Disability Concept." *Hypatia* 26.3 (2014): 591–609.

Garland-Thomson, Rosemarie. "Siri and Me." *Huffington Post*, September 2, 2013; accessed November 14, 2016.

Gidney, Catherine. *Tending the Student Body: Youth, Health, and the Modern University*. Toronto: University of Toronto Press, 2015.

Giroux, Henry. *Neoliberalism's War on Higher Education*. Chicago: Haymarket Books, 2014.

Gleeson, Brendan. *Geographies of Disability*. New York: Routledge, 1999.

Goddard, Henry H. "Mental Tests and the Immigrant." *Journal of Delinquency* 2 (1917): 243–77.

Goffman, Erving. "On the Characteristics of Total Institutions." *Symposium on Preventive and Social Psychiatry*. Washington, DC: Walter Reed Army Medical Centre, 1961.

Goggin, Gerard, and Christopher Newell. "Disabling Cell Phones." *The Cell Phone Reader: Essays in Social Transformation*, edited by Anandam P. Kavoori and Noah Arceneaux, 155–72. London: Peter Lang, 2006.

Goldrick-Rab, Sara, Katharine Broton, and Daniel Eisenberg. "Hungry to learn: Addressing food and housing insecurity among undergraduates." *Wisconsin Hope Lab* (2015).

Graff, Harvey J. *Literacy Myths, Legacies, and Lessons: New Studies on Literacy*. New York: Transaction Publishers, 2011.

Grasgreen, Allie. "Students with Disabilities Frustrated with Ignorance and Lack of Services." *Inside Higher Education*, April 2, 2014; accessed November 1, 2016.

Grego, Rhonda, and Nancy Thompson. "Repositioning Remediation: Renegotiating Composition's Work in the Academy." *College Composition and Communication* 47.1 (1996): 62–84.

Grace, Elizabeth. "Cognitively Accessible Language (Why We Should Care)." *Feminist Wire* 2013; accessed March 10, 2016.

Greene, Thomas G., C. Nathan Marti, and Kay McClenney. "The Effort-Outcome Gap: Differences for African American and Hispanic Community College Students in Student Engagement and Academic Achievement." *Journal of Higher Education* 79.5 (2008): 513–39.

Gugerty, John. "An Investigation of Factors Associated with Degree Completion." University of Wisconsin Center on Education and Work, 2005.

Gutiérrez y Muhs, Gabriella, Yolanda Flores Niemann, Carmen Gonzalez, and Angela P. Harris, eds. *Presumed Incompetent: The Intersections of Race and Class for Women in Academia.* Boulder: University Press of Colorado, 2012.

Halberstam, Judith. *The Queer Art of Failure.* Durham, NC: Duke University Press, 2011.

Hamraie, Aimi. "Designing Collective Access." *DSQ* 33.4 (2013).

Harbour, Wendy S. *Final Report: The 2004 AHEAD Survey of Higher Education Disability Services Providers.* Huntersville, NC: Association of Higher Education and Disability, 2004.

"Hard-of-Hearing Alumna Outraged at University's Lack of Action, Again." *CBC News,* September 18, 2015; accessed November 1, 2016.

Hardt, Michael, and Antonio Negri. *Multitude: War and Democracy in the Age of Empire.* New York: Penguin Press, 2004.

Harris, Malcolm. "Reform School." *New Inquiry,* March 18, 2016; accessed November 1, 2016.

Harrison, Allyson G., and Joan Wolforth. "Findings from a pan-Canadian survey of disability services providers in post-secondary education." *International Journal of Disability, Community & Rehabilitation* 11.1 (2012): 1–39.

Harvey, David. "From Space to Place and Back Again: Reflections on the Condition of Postmodernity." In *Mapping the Futures: Local Cultures, Global Change,* edited by Jon Bird. London: Routledge, 1993.

Harvey, David. "Neoliberalism as Creative Destruction." *Annals of the American Academy of Political and Social Science* 610.1 (2007): 21–44.

Havighurst, Walter. *The Miami Years, 1809–1969.* New York: Putnam, 1969.

Hawisher, Gail E., et al. "Becoming literate in the information age: Cultural ecologies and the literacies of technology." *College Composition and Communication* (2004): 642–92.

Hawisher, Gail E., and Cynthia L. Selfe. "2014 CCCC Exemplar Award Acceptance Speech." *College Composition and Communication* 67.1 (2015): 121.

Healy, Kieran. "*Monsters University*: The Aftermath." https://kieranhealy.org/blog/archives/2013/06/22/monsters-university-the-aftermath/

Helquist, Melissa. "Eye, Hand, Ear: Multimodal Literacy Practices of Blind Adults." PhD diss., Texas Tech University, 2105.

Hendren, Sara, and Caitlyn Lynch. "Manifesto: Engineering at Home." *Engineering at Home,* January 1, 2016; accessed March 10, 2016.

Higbee, J. L., D. B. Lundell, H. L. Barajas, R.J. Cordano, and R. Copeland. "Implementing Universal Instructional Design: Resources for Faculty." Presentation at the 22nd Annual Pacific Rim Conference on Disabilities, Honolulu, March 2006.

Higher Education Statistical Agency. *Yearly Overviews,* January 12, 2017; accessed February 19, 2006.

Hiltzik, Michael. "Does Congress Have the Heart to Avert Disability Crisis?" *Los Angeles Times,* February 2, 2013; accessed November 14, 2016.

Hirschman, Albert O. *The Rhetoric of Reaction.* Cambridge: Harvard University Press, 1991.

Hitt, Allison. "Access for All: The Role of Dis/ability in Multiliteracy Centers." *Praxis: A Writing Center Journal* 9.2 (2012).

Hoffman, Claire. "The Battle for Facebook." *Rolling Stone*, June 28, 2008; accessed February 5, 2009.

Holmes, M. Morgan. "Big Promises, Bigger Failures: When Public Education Makes You Sick." *Nursing Clio*, August 27, 2015; accessed March 1, 2016.

Horner, Bruce, and Min-Zhan Lu. *Representing the "Other": Basic Writers and the Teaching of Basic Writing.* Urbana, IL: National Council for Teachers of English Press, 1992.

Hornstein, Gail A. "Why I Dread the Accommodations Talk." *The Chronicle of Higher Education.* N.p., 26 Mar. 2017. Web. 28 Mar. 2017.

Howard-Jones, Paul A. "Neuroscience and Education: Myths and Messages." *Nature Reviews Neuroscience* 15.12 (2014): 817–24.

Howe, Henry. *Historical Collections of Ohio: In Two Volumes. An Encyclopedia of the State.* Vol. 1. Columbus: State of Ohio, 1907.

Hsu, Hua. "The Year of the Imaginary College Student." *New Yorker*, March 31, 2015; accessed November 14, 2016.

Hunter, Daniel G. "Out of Sight, Out of Mind: Disability and the Aesthetics of Landscape Architecture." *Adaptive Environments* (May 1999).

"If Hogwarts' Houses Were Ivy League Schools." *Ivy League Lifestyle*, February 23, 2015; accessed March 10, 2016.

Imrie, Rob. "Access in the Built Environment." In *The Disability Reader: Social Science Perspectives*, edited by Tom Shakespeare, 129–147. London: Cassell, 1998.

"In Academia, There Is No Such Thing as Winning a Sexual Harassment Complaint." *Guardian*, August 9, 2013; accessed November 1, 2016.

Istvan, Zoltan. "In the Transhumanist Age, We Should Be Repairing Disabilities, Not Sidewalks." *Motherboard.Vice.com*, March 10, 2016.

Jack, Jordynn. "What Are Neurorhetorics?" *Rhetoric Society Quarterly* 40.5 (2010): 405–10.

Jacobs, Peter. "The Real Life Buildings That Helped Inspire the *Monsters University* Campus." *Business Insider*, July 2, 2013. http://www.businessinsider.com/buildings-inspire-monsters-university-2013-7

Jacobs, Steve. "The Electronic Curb-Cut Effect." Developed in support of the *World Bank Conference: Disability and Development.* Duluth, GA: NCR Corporation, 1999.

Jaschik, Scott. "Rudy Giuliani: Students Who Protest Are 'Crybabies'." *Inside Higher Education*, November 12, 2016.

Jay, Martin. "Photo-Unrealism: The Contribution of the Camera to the Crisis of Ocularcentrism." In *Vision and Textuality*, 344–60. London: Macmillan Education UK, 1995.

Johnson, Mary. *Make Them Go Away: Clint Eastwood, Christopher Reeve, and the Case against Disability Rights.* Louisville, KY: Advocado Press, 2003.

Johnson, Robert R. *User-Centered Technology: A Rhetorical Theory for Computers and Other Mundane Artifacts.* Albany: SUNY Press, 1998.

Johnstone, Marjorie, and Eunjung Lee. "Branded: International Education and 21st-Century Canadian Immigration, Education Policy, and the Welfare State." *International Social Work* 57.3 (2014): 209–21.

Jones, Richard. "Miami Students May Face Charges for Rape Flier." *Journal-News.com*, October 23, 2012; accessed March 8, 2016.

Joost, Gesche, Tom Bieling. "Design against Normality." *V!RUS* 7 (2012).

Kafer, Alison. *Feminist Queer Crip.* Bloomington: Indiana University Press, 2013.

Keates, Simeon, and John Clarkson. "Countering Design Exclusion." In *Inclusive Design*, by Simeon Keates and John Clarkson, 438–53. London: Springer London,

2003.Keely, Karen A. "Madcap Eugenics in College Holiday." In *Popular Eugenics: National Efficiency and American Mass Culture in the 1930s*, edited by Susan Currell. Athens: Ohio University Press, 2006.

Kelty, Christopher, Michael M. J. Fisher, Alex Golub, Jason Baird Johnson, et al. "Anthropology of/in Circulation: The Future of Open Access and Scholarly Societies." *Cultural Anthropology* 23.3 (2008): 559–88.

Kendall, Connie. "Nooses and Neck Verses: The Life and Death Consequences of Literacy Testing." *Rhetorical Agendas: Political, Ethical, Spiritual* (2006): 97.

Kendall, Lori. "Nerd Nation Images of Nerds in US Popular Culture." *International Journal of Cultural Studies* 2.2 (1999): 260–83.

Kerschbaum, Stephanie L. *Toward a New Rhetoric of Difference*. Urbana, IL: Conference on College Composition and Communication/National Council of Teachers of English, 2014.

Kerschbaum, Stephanie, and Jay Dolmage. "Wanted: Disabled Faculty." *Inside Higher Education*, November 1, 2016; accessed November 5, 2016.

Kerschbaum, Stephanie, and Margaret Price. "Perils and Prospects of Disclosing Disability Identity in Higher Education." Blog post, March 2014, http://sites.udel.edu/csd/2014/03/03/perils-and-prospects-of-disclosing-disabilityidentity-in-higher-education.

Kiley, Kevin. "College Is Scary." *Inside Higher Ed*, June 21, 2013; http://www.insidehighered.com/news/2013/06/21/monsters-university-explores-value-diversity-college-settings#ixzz2h3vbRp5f

King, J. C. H. *Blood and Land: The Story of Native North America*. New York: Allen Lane, 2016.

Kingma, Boris, and Wouter van Marken Lichtenbelt. "Energy Consumption in Buildings and Female Thermal Demand." *Nature Climate Change* (August 2015).

Kinkade, Patrick T., and Michael A. Katovich. "Toward a Sociology of Cult Films: Reading *Rocky Horror*." *Sociological Quarterly* 33 (1992): 191–209.

Kinman, Gail, and Siobhan Wray. "Higher Stress: A Survey of Stress and Well-Being among Staff in Higher Education." University and College Union report, July 2013. https://www.ucu.org.uk/media/5911/Higher-stress-a-survey-of-stress-and-well-being-among-staff-in-higher-education-Jul-13/pdf/HE_stress_report_July_2013.pdf

Kirkham, Chris. "For-Profit College Recruiters Taught To Use 'Pain,' 'Fear,' Internal Documents Show." *Huffington Post*, March 10, 2016.

Kliewer, Christopher, Douglas Biklen, and Christi Kasa-Hendrickson. "Who May Be Literate? Disability and Resistance to the Cultural Denial of Competence." *American Educational Research Journal* 43.2 (2006): 163–92.

Kobayashi, Audrey. "Critical 'Race' Approaches to Cultural Geography." In *A Companion to Cultural Geography*, edited by James S. Duncan, Nuala C. Johnson, and Richard H. Schein, 238–49. London: Wiley, 2004.

Kodak Corp. *A Brief History of Design & Usability at Kodak*. Accessed June 24, 2005.

Konrad, Annika. "Access as a Lens for Peer Tutoring." *Another Word*, February 22, 2016; accessed November 1, 2016.

Kress, Gunther. "Genres and the multimodal production of 'scientificness'." *Multimodal Literacy* (2003): 173–86.

Kress, Gunther. *Multimodality: A Social Semiotic Approach to Contemporary Communication*. New York: Routledge, 2009.

Kress, Gunther, and Theo Van Leeuwen. *Multimodal Discourse: The Modes and Media of Contemporary Communication*. London: Edward Arnold, 2001.

Krisch, Joshua A. "When Racism Was a Science." *New York Times*, October 13, 2014; accessed November 11, 2016.

Krueger, Sarah, Jennifer Obinna, Constance Osterbaan, Jane M. Sadusky, and Wendy DeVore. *Understanding the Needs of the Victims of Sexual Assault in the Deaf Community: A Needs Assessment and Audit.* New York: Council on Crime and Justice, 2005. https://www.ncjrs.gov/pdffiles1/nij/grants/212867.pdf

Krupnick, Matt. "Colleges Respond to Growing Ranks of Learning Disabled." *Washington Monthly* (February 2014): 1–4.

Kudlick, Catherine, and Susan Schweik. "Collision and Collusion: Artists, Academics, and Activists in Dialogue with the University of California and Critical Disability Studies." *Disability Studies Quarterly* 34.2 (2014).

Kumari Campbell, Fiona. *Contours of Ableism: The Production of Disability and Abledness.* London: Palgrave Macmillan, 2009.

Kuusisto, Stephen. "Disability, the Academy, and Gestural Violence." *Planet of the Blind,* March 26, 2015; accessed March 10, 2016.

Kuusisto, Stephen. "Higher Education's Studied Indifference to People with Disabilities Reflects the "Rehab Model" Ad Nauseum." *Planet of the Blind,* July 19, 2009; accessed March 10, 2016.

Lanham, Richard A. *The Economics of Attention: Style and Substance in the Age of Information.* Chicago: University of Chicago Press, 2006.

Laughlin, Henry. "Report of H.H Laughlin for the Year Ending August 31, 1922." Charles B. Davenport Papers, American Philosophical Society.

Lefebvre, Henri. "The Right to the City." In *Writings on Cities,* edited by Eleonore Kofman and Elizabeth Lebas, 63–181. London: Wiley-Blackwell, 1996.

Le Feuvre, Lisa. "Art Failure." *Art Monthly* 313.2 (2008): 5–8.

Leland L., Glenna, Margaret A. Gollnick, and Stephen S. Jones. "Eugenic Opportunity Structures: Teaching Genetic Engineering at US Land-Grant Universities since 1911."*Social Studies of Science* 37.2 (April 2007): 281–96.

Lewiecki-Wilson, Cynthia. "Rethinking *Rhetoric* through Mental *Disabilities.*" *Rhetoric Review* 22.2 (2003): 154–202.

Linden, Myra J., and Arthur Whimbey. *Why Johnny Can't Write: How to Improve Writing Skills.* New York: Routledge, 2012.

Linton, Simi. "Reassigning Meaning." In *Claiming Disability: Knowledge and Identity,* 8–33. New York: NYU Press, 1993.

"The Little Girl Who Crawled up the Capitol Steps 25 Years Later: Jennifer Keelan and the ADA." *Cerebral Palsy Daily Living,* July 29, 2015; accessed November 11, 2016.

Lo Bianco, Joseph. "National Space and Linguistic Borders." Presented at the Tenth International Colloquium on "Problems and Methods in the History of Languages," University of Girona, Girona, Spain, June 27–29, 2016. Long, Elenore. "Rhetorical Techne, Local Knowledge, and Challenges in Contemporary Activism." *Rhetorics, Literacies, and Narratives of Sustainability* 1 (2009): 13.

Looker, E. D., and G. S. Lowe. "Post-secondary Access and Student Financial Aid in Canada: Current Knowledge and Research Gaps." Ottawa, ON: Canadian Policy Research Networks, 2001.

Losen, Daniel J., and Jonathan Gillespie. "Opportunities Suspended: The Disparate Impact of Disciplinary Exclusion from School." Los Angeles: Civil Rights Project, University of California at Los Angeles, 2012.

Lucchesi, Anderw J. "Accessing Academe, Disabling the Curriculum: Institutional Locations of Dis/ability in Public Higher Education." PhD diss., City University of New York, 2016.

Mace, Ronald L. "Universal Design, Barrier Free Environments for Everyone." *Designers West* 33.1 (1985): 147–52.

MacFarlane, Bruce. "Academic Double Standards: Freedom for Lecturers, Compliance for Students." *Times Higher Education*, September 28, 2016; accessed October 31, 2016.

Mackey, Eva. *House of Difference: Cultural Politics and National Identity in Canada.* London: Routledge, 1999.

Mallick, Heather. "Why Keep Mental Disability a Secret?" *Toronto Star*, January 15, 2016; accessed November 14, 2016. https://www.thestar.com/news/gta/2016/01/15/why-keep-mental-disability-a-secret-mallick.html

Manning, Erin, and Brian Massumi. *Thought in the Act: Passages in the Ecology of Experience.* Minneapolis: University of Minnesota Press, 2014.

Marback, Richard. "The Rhetorical Space of Robben Island." *Rhetoric Society Quarterly* 34.2 (2004): 7–27.

Maroto, M. "Food Insecurity among Community College Students: Prevalence and Relationship to GPA, Energy, and Concentration." PhD diss., Morgan State University, 2013.

Maroto, M. E., A. Snelling, and H. Linck. "Food Insecurity among Community College Students: Prevalence and Association with Grade Point Average." *Community College Journal of Research and Practice* 39.6 (2015): 515–26.

Martin, Emily. *Bipolar Expeditions: Mania and Depression in American Culture.* Princeton: Princeton University Press, 2007.

McCarthy, Cameron, Alicia P. Rodriguez, Ed Buendia, Shuaib Meacham, Stephen David, Heriberto Godina, K. E. Supriya, and Carrie Wilson-Brown. "Danger in the Safety Zone: Notes on Race, Resentment, and the Discourse of Crime, Violence and Suburban Security." *Cultural Studies* 11.2 (1997): 274–95.

McGill University. "Universal Design." *Mcgill.ca*, March 7, 2016.

McLaren, Angus. *Our Own Master Race: Eugenics in Canada, 1885–1945.* Toronto: University of Toronto Press, 2015.

McLean, Patricia, Margaret Heagney, and Kay Gardner. "Going Global: The Implications for Students with a Disability." *Higher Education Research and Development* 22.2 (2003): 217–28.

Melnick, Jeffrey, and Rachel Rubin. *Immigration and American Popular Culture: An Introduction* New York: NYU Press, 2007.

Metzel, Deborah S., and Pamela M. Walker. "The Illusion of Inclusion: Geographies of the Lives of People with Developmental Disabilities in the United States." *Disability Studies Quarterly* 21.4 (2001): 114–28.

"Miami Mergers Are Part of University's Conscious Coupling." *NY Daily News*, April 1, 2014; accessed March 7, 2016.

Michalko, Rod, and Tanya Titchkosky. "Putting Disability in Its Place: It's Not a Joking Matter." In *Embodied Rhetorics: Disability in Language and Culture*, edited by James C. Wilson and Cynthia Lewiecki-Wilson, 200–28. Carbondale: Southern Illinois University Press, 2001.

Mills, Mara. "Hearing Aids and the History of Electronics Miniaturization." *Annals of the History of Computing, IEEE* 33.2 (2011): 24–45.

Mingus, Mia. "Access Intimacy: The Missing Link." *Leaving Evidence*, May 5, 2011; accessed November 1, 2016.

Miranda, Melinna. "Police Carding Affects Racialized Students on University Campuses, Activists Say." *Ryersonian.ca*, February 24, 2016; accessed March 2, 2016.

Mitchell, David T., and Sharon L. Snyder. *The Biopolitics of Disability.* University of Michigan Press,, 2015.

Mitchell, David T. "Disability, Diversity, and Diversion." In *Disability, Avoidance and the*

Academy: Challenging Resistance, edited by David Bolt and Claire Penketh, 9. London: Taylor and Francis, 2015. 9–33.

Mitchell, Jerry. "Graves' Discovery Affects Miss. Medical School's Plans." *Jackson* (MS) *Clarion-Ledger,* February 9, 2014; http://www.usatoday.com/story/news/nation/2014/02/09/mississippi-medical-school-graves-found/5320995/

Mitra, Shayoni. "'It Takes Six People to Make a Mattress Feel Light . . .': Materializing Pain in Carry That Weight and Sexual Assault Activism." *Contemporary Theatre Review* 25.3 (2015): 386–400.

Mohamed, Sarah. "Student Loans a Major Source of Discrimination against Post-Secondary Students with Disabilities." *BakerLaw,* June 16, 2014; accessed March 10, 2016.

Moodley, Roy. "Multi (ple) Cultural Voices Speaking 'Outside the Sentence' of Counselling and Psychotherapy." *Counselling Psychology Quarterly* 22.3 (2009): 297–307.

Mosby, Ian. "Administering Colonial Science: Nutrition Research and Human Biomedical Experimentation in Aboriginal Communities and Residential Schools, 1942–1952." *Histoire sociale/Social history* 46.1 (2013): 145–72. Accessed online at *Project MUSE,* June 1, 2015.

Mountford, Roxanne. "On Gender and Rhetorical Space." *Rhetoric Society Quarterly* 31.1 (2001): 41–71.

Murphy, Michelle. *Sick Building Syndrome and the Problem of Uncertainty: Environmental Politics, Technoscience, and Women Workers.* Durham, NC: Duke University Press, 2006.

Murray, Charles. "The Coming Apart of America's Civic Culture." *Journal of Research in Character Education* 10.1 (2014): 1.

Murray, Joddy. *Non-discursive Rhetoric: Image and Affect in Multimodal Composition.* Albany, NY: SUNY Press, 2009.

"Nasty e-mail, cross burning irk Miami." *Cincinnati Enquirer.* N.p., 31 Oct. 2002. Web. 09 Mar. 2017. N.p., 31 Oct. 2002. Web. 09 Mar. 2017.

National Center for Education Statistics. "Fast Facts: Students with Disabilities." Washington: U.S Department of Education, 2016.

National Lampoon's Animal House. Dir. John Landis. Universal, 1978.

North Carolina State University. "Center for Universal Design: Principles of Universal Design, Version 2.0." Raleigh: Center for Universal Design, North Carolina State University, 1997.

Nguyen, Mary. "Degreeless in Debt: What Happens to Borrowers Who Drop Out. Charts You Can Trust." Washington, DC: Education Sector, 2012.

O'Hearn, Carolyn. "Recognizing the Learning Disabled College Writer." *College English* 51.3 (1989): 294–304.

Ohio State University Partnership Grant Improving the Quality of Education for Students with Disabilities. "Fast Facts for Faculty: Universal Design for Learning, Elements of Good Teaching." http://telr.osu.edu/dpg/fastfact/fastfactcolor/Universal.pdf

Oliver, Michael. *Understanding Disability: From Theory to Practice.* New York: St Martin's, 1996.

Olney, Marjorie F., & Amanda Kim. "Beyond adjustment: Integration of Cognitive Disability into Identity." *Disability & Society* 16 (2001): 563–83.

Onion, Rebecca. "Take the Impossible 'Literacy' Test Louisiana Gave Black Voters in the 1960s." *Slate.com,* June 28, 2003; accessed February 29, 2016.

Oparah, Julia. "Challenging Complicity: The Neoliberal University and the Prison-Industrial Complex." In *The Imperial University: Academic Repression and Scholarly*

Dissent, edited by Piya Chatterjee and Sunaina Maira. Minneapolis: University of Minnesota Press, 2014.

Orchowski, Lindsay M., Brad A. Spickard, and John R. McNamara. "Cinema and the Valuing of Psychotherapy: Implications for Clinical Practice." *Professional Psychology: Research and Practice* 37.5 (2006): 506.

Ordover, Nancy. "American Eugenics." In *Race, Queer Anatomy, and the Science of Nationalism.* Minneapolis: University of Minnesota Press, 2003.

Orem, Sarah, and Neil Simpkins. "Weepy Rhetoric, Trigger Warnings, and the Work of Making Mental Illness Visible in the Writing Classroom." *Enculturation,* March 10, 2015; accessed November 14, 2016.

Organisation for Economic Co-Operation and Development (OECD). *Education at a Glance 2011: OECD Indicators.* Paris: OECD, 2010.

Orr, David. "Architecture as Pedagogy." In *Reshaping the Built Environment: Ecology, Ethics, and Economics,* edited by Charles J. Kilbert, 212–18. Washington, DC: Island Press, 1999.

O'Shea, Amber, and Rachel H. Meyer. "A Qualitative Investigation of the Motivation of College Students with Nonvisible Disabilities to Utilize Disability Services." *Journal of Postsecondary Education and Disability* 29.1 (2016): 5–23.

Oswal, Sushil. "Ableism." In "Multimodality in Motion: Disability and Kairotic Spaces," a special issue edited by Melanie Yergeau et al. *Kairos: A Journal of Rhetoric, Technology, and Pedagogy* 18.1 (August 2013).

Oswal, Sushil K., Stephanie L. Kerschbaum, Rosemarie Garland-Thomson, Amy Vidali, et al. "Faculty Members, Accommodation, and Access in Higher Education." *Profession* (2013).https://profession.mla.hcommons.org/2013/12/09/faculty-members-accommodation-and-access-in-higher-education/

Porter, James E., Patricia Sullivan, Stuart Blythe, Jeffrey T. Grabill, and Libby Miles. "Institutional Critique: A Rhetorical Methodology for Change." *College Composition and Communication* 51.4 (2000): 610–42.

Postgraduate. "In Academia, There Is No Such Thing as Winning a Sexual Harassment Complaint." *Guardian,* February 9, 2013; accessed November 14, 2016.

Powell, Pegeen Reichert. "Retention and Writing Instruction: Implications for Access and Pedagogy." *College Composition and Communication* (2009): 664–82.

Prescott, Heather Munro. *Student Bodies: The Influence of Student Health Services in American Society and Medicine.* Ann Arbor: University of Michigan Press, 2007.

Price, Margaret. "Access: A Happening." Featured session, in collaboration with Jay Dolmage, Qwo-Li Driskill, Cynthia Selfe, et al. Conference on College Composition and Communication. St. Louis, MO. March 23, 2012.

Price, Margaret. "It Shouldn't Be So Hard." *Inside Higher Ed* 7 (2011).

Price, Margaret. *Mad at School: Rhetorics of Mental Disability and Academic Life.* Ann Arbor: University of Michigan Press, 2011.

Pryal, Katie Rose Guest. "The Creativity Mystique and the Rhetoric of Mood Disorders." *Disability Studies Quarterly* 31.3 (2011): n.p. http://dsq-sds.org/article/view/1671/1600

Puar, Jasbir K. "Coda: The Cost of Getting Better: Suicide, Sensation, Switchpoints." *GLQ: A Journal of Lesbian and Gay Studies* 18.1 (2012): 149–58.

Pullin, Graham. *Design Meets Disability.* Cambridge, MA: MIT Press, 2009.

Quigley, Margaret. "The Roots of the I.Q. Debate: Eugenics and Social Control." *The Public Eye,* 1995. http://www.hartford-hwp.com/archives/45/034.html

Ratner, Romesh. "Lost in the Middle." *Time,* March 24, 2001; accessed November 12, 2016.

Read, Jacinda. "The Cult of Masculinity: From Fan-Boys to Academic Bad-Boys." In

Defining Cult Movies: The Cultural Politics of Oppositional Tastes, edited by Mark Jancovich. Manchester: Manchester University Press, 2003.

Reichert, Pegeen Powell. *Retention and Resistance: Writing Instruction and Students Who Leave*. Logan: Utah State University Press, 2013.

Riedner, Rachel C. *Writing Neoliberal Values: Rhetorical Connectivities and Globalized Capitalism*. New York: Springer, 2015.

Rensselaer Polytechnic Institute Library Archives. "The Approach." http://www.lib. rpi.edu/dept/library/html/Archives/gallery/approach/apphome.html

Richter, Zach. "Some Notes on Communication Accessibility: A Term Just Now Finding Life." *Did I Stutter*, 2015; http://didistutterproject.tumblr.com/post/135447707437/some-notes-on-communication-accessibility-a-term

Ridolfo, Jim, and Dànielle Nicole DeVoss. "Composing for Recomposition: Rhetorical Velocity and Delivery." *Kairos: A Journal of Rhetoric, Technology, and Pedagogy* 13.2 (2009): n2. http://kairos.technorhetoric.net/13.2/topoi/ridolfo_devoss/

Robbins, Bruce. "Celeb-Reliance: Intellectuals, Celebrity, and Upward Mobility." *Postmodern Culture* 9.2 (1999).Rose, Marilyn. Accommodating graduate students with disabilities. Council of Ontario Universities, 2010.

Rosenfeld, Arno. "Company Town: How Campus Became Commercial." *Ubyssey*, October 19, 2015; accessed November 10, 2016.

Ross, Andrew. *No Respect: Intellectuals and Popular Culture*. London: Routledge, 2016.

Rothman, David J. *The Discovery of the Asylum*. New York: Transaction Publishers, 1971.

Rothman, Joshua. "Why Is Academic Writing So Academic?" *New Yorker*,February 20, 2014; accessed November 14, 2016.Sailor, Wayne, and Matt Stowe. "School Vouchers and Students with Disabilities. Policy Paper." National Council on Disability. (2003).

Samuels, Ellen. *Fantasies of Identification: Disability, Gender, Race*. New York: NYU Press, 2014.

Sandage, Scott A. *Born Losers*. Cambridge: Harvard University Press, 2005.

Saul, John Ralston. *The Comeback: How Aboriginals Are Reclaiming Power and Influence*. Toronto: Penguin Canada, 2014.

Schick, Carol. "Keeping the Ivory Tower White: Discourses ot Racial Domination." *Canadian Journal of Law and Society* 15.2 (2000): 70–90.

Schweik, Susan M. *The Ugly Laws: Disability in Public*. New York: NYU Press, 2009.

Scott, Jerrie Cobb, Dolores Y. Straker, and Laurie Katz, eds. *Affirming Students' Right to Their Own Language: Bridging Language Policies and Pedagogical Practices*. New York: Routledge, 2009.

Sedlacek, William E. "Using Noncognitive Variables in Assessing Readiness for Higher Education." *Readings on Equal Education* 25 (2011): 187–205.

Selber, Stuart. *Multiliteracies for a Digital Age*. Carbondale: Southern Illinois University Press, 2004.

Selfe, Cynthia L. Ed. *Multimodal Composition: Resources for Teachers*. Boston: Hampton Press, 2007.

Selfe, Cynthia L. *Technology and literacy in the 21st century: The importance of paying attention*. SIU Press, 1999.

Selfe, Cynthia, and Richard Selfe. "The Politics of the Interface." *CCC* 45.4 (1994): 480–503.

Serlin, David. *Replaceable You: Engineering the Body in Postwar America*. Chicago: University of Chicago Press, 2004.

Shalit, Ruth. "Defining Disability Down." *New Republic* 40 (1997): 16–27.

Shakespeare, Tom. "Rules of Engagement: Doing Disability Research." *Disability & Society* 11.1 (1996): 115–21.

Shapiro, Joseph. *No Pity: People with Disabilities Forging a New Civil Rights Movement.* New York: Random House, 1993.

Sharav, Vera Hassner. "Human Experiments: A Chronology of Human Research." *Alliance for Human Research Protection,* December 8, 2004; http://www.research-protection.org/history/chronology.html

Shigaki, Cheryl L., et al. "Disability on Campus: A Perspective from Faculty and Staff." *Work* 42.4 (2012): 559–71.

Sibley, David. *Geographies of Exclusion: Society and Difference in the West.* New York: Routledge, 1995.

Siebers, Tobin. *Disability Theory.* Ann Arbor: University of Michigan Press, 2010.

Silva, Steve. "MSVU Student Not Allowed to Tell Others He's Suicidal per School's Wellness Agreement." *Global News,* May 16, 2016; accessed November 1, 2016.

Silverthorn, D. "Hungry for Knowledge: Assessing the Prevalence of Student Food Insecurity on Five Canadian Campuses." Toronto: Meal Exchange, 2016.

Slaughter, Sheila, and Larry L. Leslie. *Academic Capitalism: Politics, Policies, and the Entrepreneurial University.* Baltimore: Johns Hopkins University Press, 1997.

Smith, S. E. "Why Are Huge Numbers of Disabled Students Dropping Out of College?" *Alternet,* March 20, 2014; accessed March 10, 2016.

Snyder, Sharon L., and David T. Mitchell. "Body Genres: An Anatomy of Disability in Film." In *The Problem Body: Projecting Disability on Film,* edited by Sally Chivers and Nicole Markotiⵜ, 179–204. Columbus: Ohio State University Press, 2010.

Snyder, Sharon L., and David T. Mitchell. *Cultural Locations of Disability.* Chicago: University of Chicago Press, 2010.

Snyder, Sharon L., and David T. Mitchell. *Narrative Prosthesis: Disability and the Dependence of Discourse.* Ann Arbor: University of Michigan Press, 2001.

Snyder, Sharon L., and David T. Mitchell. "Re-engaging the Body: Disability Studies and the Resistance to Embodiment." *Public Culture* 13.3 (2001): 367–89.

Snyder, Sharon L., and David T. Mitchell. "Representation and Its Discontents: The Uneasy Home of Disability in Literature and Film." In *Handbook of Disability Studies,* edited by G. L. Albrecht, K. D. Seelman, and M. Bury, 195–218. Thousand Oaks, CA: Sage Publications, 2001.

Sokal, Laura. "ETTA Use in Canadian Postsecondary Schools." *Canadian Journal of Disability Studies* 5.3 (December 2016).

Sokolower, Jody. "Schools and the New Jim Crow: An Interview with Michelle Alexander." *Rethinking Schools* (Winter 2012).

Somerville, Siobhan B. *Queering the Color Line: Race and the Invention of Homosexuality in American Culture.* Durham, NC: Duke University Press, 2000.

Soorenian, Armineh. "The Significance of Studying Disabled International Students' Experiences in UK Universities." In *The Disability Press.* Leeds, UK: Centre for Disability Studies, University of Leeds, 2008.

Statistics Canada. "Canadian Survey on Disability." Ottawa: 2012.

Steele, Claude M. "Race and the Schooling of Black Americans." *Atlantic Monthly* 269.4 (1992): 68–78.

Steinfeld, Edward, and Jordana Maisel. *Universal Design: Creating Inclusive Environments.* New York: John Wiley and Sons, 2012.

Stender, Lisa. "Trouble with Classes? Mountaineer Academic Program Provides Academic Coaching, Tutoring." *Diversity.wvu.edu,* July 21, 2014; accessed March 7, 2016.

Sternberg, Robert. "Everything's an Illness." *New York Times,* August 31, 1997; accessed November 14, 2016.

Story, Molly Follette. "Maximizing Usability: The Principles of Universal Design." *Assistive Technology* 10.1 (1998): 4–12.

St. Pierre, Joshua, and Danielle Peers. "Telling Ourselves Sideways, Crooked and Crip: An Introduction." *Canadian Journal of Disability Studies* 5.3 (2016): 1–11.

Stramondo, Joseph. "The Medicalization of Reasonable Accommodation." *Discrimination and Disadvantage*, January 31, 2015; accessed November 1, 2016.

Strauss, Valerie. "The telling letter Betsy DeVos wrote to clarify her position on U.S. disabilities law." *The Washington Post*. 28 Jan. 2017. Web. 24 Mar. 2017.

Street, Steve, Maria Maisto, Esther Merves, and Gary Rhoades. (2013). "Who Is Professor 'Staff'? *Center for the Future of Higher Education* Policy Report 2 (August 2012).1–22.

Strickland, Donna. *The Managerial Unconscious in the History of Composition Studies.* Carbondale, IL: SIU Press, 2011.

Stubblefield, Anna. ""Beyond the Pale": Tainted Whiteness, Cognitive Disability, and Eugenic Sterilization." *Hypatia* 22.2 (2007): 162–81.

Stuckey, J. Elspeth. *The Violence of Literacy.* Portsmouth, NH: Boynton/Cook Publishers, 1991.

Stuckey, Zosha. *A Rhetoric of Remnants: Idiots, Half-wits, and Other State-Sponsored Inventions.* Albany: SUNY Press, 2014.

Stuckey, Zosha, and Lois P. Agnew. "Rhetoric, Ethos, and Unease: Re-negotiation of the 'Normal' in the Classroom and on the Quad." *Open Words: Access and English Studies* 5 (2011): 15–28.

Stuckler, David, and Sanjay Basu. *The Body Economic: Why Austerity Kills.* London: Allen Lane, 2013.

Suber, Peter, Patrick O. Brown, Diane Cabell, Aravinda Chakravarti, Barbara Cohen, Tony Delamothe, Michael Eisen et al. *Bethesda Statement on Open Access Publishing.* 2003. http://www.earlham.edu/~peters/fos/bethesda.htm

Sullivan, Patricia. "Feminism and Methodology in Composition Studies." In *Methods and Methodology in Composition Research*, edited by Patricia A. Sullivan and Gesa E. Kirsch. Carbondale: Southern Illinois University Press, 1992

Taylor, Astra. "Universities Are Becoming Billion-Dollar Hedge Funds with Schools Attached." *Nation*, March 8, 2016; accessed March 8, 2016.

Taylor and Francis. "Alternative Format Requests." 2014. http://www.taylorandfrancis.com/info/viprequests/

Thompson, Terry, Sheryl Burgstahler, Elizabeth Moore, Jon Gunderson, and Nicholas Hoyt. "International Research on Web Accessibility for Persons with Disabilities." In *Managing Worldwide Operations and Communications with Information Technology.* Hershey, PA: Information Resources Management Association, 2007.

Titchkosky, Tanya. "The Becoming Crisis of Disability Studies." Disability Studies Summer Institute keynote address, University of Toronto, Toronto, July 18, 2011.

Titchkosky, Tanya. "Cultural Maps: Which Way to Disability." In *Disability/Postmodernity: Embodying Disability Theory*, edited by Mairian Corker and Tom Shakespeare, 101–11. London: Continuum, 2002.

Titchkosky, Tanya. *The Question of Access: Disability, Space, Meaning.* Toronto: University of Toronto Press, 2011.

Titchkosky, Tanya. *Reading and Writing Disability Differently.* Toronto: University of Toronto Press, 2007.

Toomey, Dan, and Mary Jane Maguire. *Landmark College: A Short History of the First Twenty-Five Years.* Putney, VT: Landmark College, 2010.

Tremain, Shelley. "No Language Is Neutral, Part II: Ableist Language and Ableist

Exceptionism." *Discrimination and Disadvantage*, November 1, 2016; accessed November 8, 2016.

Trent, James W. *Inventing the Feeble Mind*. Berkeley: University of California Press, 1994.

Truth and Reconciliation Commission of Canada. *Honouring the Truth, Reconciling for the Future: Summary of the Final Report of the Truth and Reconciliation Commission of Canada*. Winnipeg: Truth and Reconciliation Commission of Canada, 2015.

Tyack, David B. *Turning Points in American Educational History*. New York: John Wiley and Sons, 1967.

UK Labour Force Survey, Quarter 2, 2012. *UK Data Service Discover*. https://discover.ukdataservice.ac.uk/series/?sn=2000026

University of Southern Mississippi, Office for Disability Assistance. "Accommodation Application." http://www.ids.usm.edu/ODA/default.htm

U.S. Census. 2008 American Community Survey; Current Population Reports, P70-117, U.S. Census Bureau, Washington, DC 2008.

U.S. Department of Education, National Center for Education Statistics. "National Survey of Postsecondary Faculty (NSOPF), 1999." NCES Report nos. 2002–151 and 2001–01. Washington, DC: NCES, 2004.

U.S. Department of Education, National Center for Education Statistics. "Students with Disabilities in Postsecondary Education: A Profile of Preparation, Participation, and Outcomes." NCES 1999–187, by Laura Horn and Jennifer Berktold. Washington, DC: NCES, 1999.

U.S. Senate Subcommittee on Disability Policy. "Americans with Disabilities Act of 1990." http://www.usdoj.gov/crt/ada/adahom1.htm

Veysey, Laurence R. *The Emergence of the American University*. Chicago: University of Chicago Press, 1966.

Vidali, Amy. "Performing the Rhetorical Freak Show: Disability, Student Writing, and College Admissions." *College English* 69.6 (July 2007): 615–41.

Vieira, Kate. "On the Social Consequences of Literacy." *Literacy in Composition Studies* 1.1 (2013): 26–32.

W3C. "Accessibility (All) Current Status." https://www.w3.org/standards/techs/accessibility#w3c_all

Waddell, Cynthia D. "US Web Accessibility Law in Depth." In *Web Accessibility: Web Standards and Regulatory Compliance*, by Jim Thatcher, Michael R. Burks, Christian Heilmann, Shawn Lawton Henry, et al., 511–44. Berkeley, CA: Apress, 2006.

Walmsley, Jan. "Normalisation, Emancipatory Research and Inclusive Research in Learning Disability." *Disability & Society* 16.2 (2001): 187–205.

Walpole, M., and J. Chaskes. "Advising New Students with Disabilities: Challenges and Opportunities." *Journal of College Orientation and Transition* 19.1 (2011): 37–49.

Wan, Amy J. *Producing Good Citizens: Literacy Training in Anxious Times*. Pittsburgh: University of Pittsburgh Press, 2014.

Ward, Lori. "Schools Reporting Zero Sexual Assaults on Campus Not Reflecting Reality, Critics, Students Say." *CBCnews*, November 23, 2015; accessed March 8, 2016.

Watkins, Evan. *Class Degrees: Smart Work, Managed Choice, and the Transformation of Higher Education*. New York: Fordham University Press, 2008.

Watkins, Evan. *Literacy Work in the Reign of Human Capital*. New York: Fordham University Press, 2015.

Welsome, Eileen. *The Plutonium Files: America's Secret Medical Experiments in the Cold War*. New York: Dial Press, 1999.

Wentz, Brian, Paul T. Jaeger, and Jonathan Lazar. "Retrofitting Accessibility: The

Legal Inequality of After-the-Fact Online Access to Persons with Disabilities in the United States." *First Monday* 16.11 (2011).

Wessel, Roger D., James A. Jones, Larry Markle, and Curt Westfall. "Retention and Graduation of Students with Disabilities: Facilitating Student Success." *Journal of Postsecondary Education and Disability* 21.3 (2009): 116–25.

Wetherbee, Ben. "The Cinematic Topos of Disability and the Example of Avatar: A Rhetorical Critique." *Ethos Review* 2.2 (2015).

Whitley, Leila, and Tiffany Page. "Sexism at the Centre: Locating the Problem of Sexual Harassment." *New Formations* 86.86 (2015): 34–53.

Wiegman, Robyn. *American Anatomies: Theorizing Race and Gender*. Durham, NC: Duke University Press, 1995.

Wilcox, Christie. "Lighting Dark: Fixing Academia's Mental Health Problem." *New Scientist*, October 10, 2014; accessed November 1, 2016.

Wilder, Craig Steven. *Ebony and Ivy*. New York: Bloomsbury Press, 2013.

Willett, Jeffrey, and Mary Jo Deegan. "Liminality and Disability: Rites of Passage and Community in Hypermodern Society." *Disability Studies Quarterly* 21.3 (2001).

Williams, Bronwyn. "Foreword." *Multimodal Composition: Resources for Teachers*. Cynthia Selfe, Ed. Boston: Hampton Press, 2007.

Williams, Jeffrey J. "Teach the University." *Pedagogy* 8.1 (2008): 25–42.

Williams, Patricia. *Seeing a Color-Blind Future*. New York: Farrar, Straus and Giroux, 1997.

Willinsky, John. 2006. *The Access Principle: The Case for Open Access to Research and Scholarship*. Cambridge, MA: MIT Press.

Winefield, Anthony H., Nicole Gillespie, Con Stough, Jagdish Dua, John Hapuarachchi, and Carolyn Boyd. "Occupational Stress in Australian University Staff: Results from a National Survey." *International Journal of Stress Management* 10.1 (2003): 51.

Wood, Marjorie, and Andrew Erwin. "The One Percent at State U." Institute for Policy Studies, May 21, 2014; accessed October 24, 2016.

Wood, Tara, Jay Dolmage, Margaret Price, and Cynthia Lewiecki-Wilson. "Moving beyond Disability 2.0 in Composition Studies." *Composition Studies* 42.2 (2014): 147.

Wood, Tara, Melissa Helquist, and Jay Dolmage. "Accommodation Addenda: Expanding Possibilities for Inclusion." *Praxis*. Forthcoming 2017.

Wood, Tara, and Shannon Madden. "Suggested Practices for Syllabus Accessibility Statements." *Kairos: A Journal of Rhetoric, Technology, and Pedagogy* 18.1 (2013). http://kairos.technorhetoric.net/praxis/tiki-index.php?page=Suggested_Practices_for_Syllabus_Accessibility_Statements World Bank. "Government expenditure on education, total (% of GDP)." 21 Mar. 2017. Web. 21 Mar. 2017.

Worth, Robert. "The Scandal of Special Ed." *Washington Monthly* 31.6 (June 1999): 34–38.

Wright, Bobby. "'For the Children of the Infidels'? American Indian Education in the Colonial Colleges." *American Indian Culture and Research Journal* 12.3 (1988): 1–14.

Yancey, Kathleen Blake. "Made Not Only in Words: Composition in a New Key." *College Composition and Communication*. 56.2 (December 2004): 297–328.

Yergeau, Melanie. "Circle Wars: Reshaping the Typical Autism Essay." *DSQ* 30.1 (Winter 2010). http://www.dsq-sds.org/article/view/1063/1222

Yergeau, Melanie, Elizabeth Brewer, et al. "Multimodality in Motion: Disability and Kairotic Spaces." *Kairos: A Journal of Rhetoric, Technology, and Pedagogy* 18.1 (August 2013). http://kairos.technorhetoric.net/18.1/coverweb/yergeau-et-al/

Yergeau, Melanie, and John Duffy. "Guest Editors' Introduction to Special Issue on Disability and Rhetoric." *DSQ* 31.3 (2011). http://dsq-sds.org/article/view/1682/1607

Yergeau, Melanie, and Paul Heilker. "Autism and Rhetoric." *College English* 73.5 (May 2011).485–97.

Young, Vershawn A., and Frankie Condon. "Introduction: Why Anti-Racist Activism? Why Now?" *Across the Disciplines* 10.3 (2013). https://wac.colostate.edu/atd/race/intro.cfm

Young Lee, Paula. "'Drown the Bunnies': Mount St. Mary's President Fires Faculty for Backlash against His 'Put a Glock to Their Heads' Freshman Retention Plan." *Salon.com*, February 10, 2016; accessed March 1, 2016.

Zarfas, D. E. "The Formation and Function of the Children's Psychiatric Research Institute, London, Ont." *Canadian Medical Association Journal* 88.4 (1963): 192–95.

Zdenek, Sean. *Reading Sounds: Closed-Captioned Media and Popular Culture.* Chicago: University of Chicago Press, 2015.

Zingrone, Frank. *The Media Symplex at the Edge of Meaning in the Age of Chaos.* New York: Hampton Press, 2004.

Index